Crises in Childbirth
Why Mothers Survive

LESSONS FROM THE CONFIDENTIAL
ENQUIRIES INTO MATERNAL DEATHS

Edited by

Daryl Dob BSc MB BS FRCA
Consultant Obstetric Anaesthetist
Chelsea and Westminster Hospital

Griselda Cooper OBE FRCA FRCOG
Senior Lecturer in Anaesthesia and Honorary Consultant Anaesthetist
Birmingham Women's Hospital

and

Anita Holdcroft MB ChB MD FRCA
Reader in Anaesthesia and Honorary Consultant Anaesthetist
Imperial College London and Chelsea and Westminster Hospital

Foreword by
Professor Philip Steer BSc MB BS MD FRCOG

Includes an Introduction by
Gwyneth Lewis MSc MRCGP FFPH FRCOG
Director, UK Confidential Enquiries into Maternal Deaths on behalf of the CEMACH

Radcliffe Publishing
Oxford • New York

Radcliffe Publishing Ltd
18 Marcham Road
Abingdon
Oxon OX14 1AA
United Kingdom

www.radcliffe-oxford.com
Electronic catalogue and worldwide online ordering facility.

British Library Cataloguing in Publication Data

A catalogue record for this book is available from the British Library.

ISBN-13: 978 1 84619 049 0

Typeset by Egan Reid, Auckland, New Zealand
Printed and bound by TJI Digital, Padstow, Cornwall

This book is dedicated to the families of the mothers who died, and to the anaesthetists who prevent maternal death, past, present and future.

Contents

Foreword

When I began my training in obstetrics, anaesthetists were not often seen on the average delivery suite. They were called only to give the general anaesthetic for the one or two Caesarean sections per week that then took place, and for one or two Caesarean hysterectomies a year. Regional anaesthesia was very uncommon and was often seen as the job of the obstetrician (as, in those days, was neonatal care).

Since then, the specialty of obstetric anaesthesia has come of age, and it is even rumoured that consultant obstetric anaesthetists now outnumber consultant obstetricians. Major advances in anaesthetic techniques and improvements in the understanding of pathophysiology have resulted in the suggestion that obstetric anaesthetists might restyle themselves as 'peripartum physicians.' This book reflects and recognises the growing input that obstetric anaesthetists have made not only in the care of normal labour in respect of analgesia, but also in the management of complications, be they medical or surgical. The reductions in maternal mortality over the last half century are an eloquent testimony to the value of the technical expertise in life support that anaesthetists bring to the management of labour complications. Many direct causes of maternal death have been substantially reduced as a result of anaesthetic innovations ranging from advances in regional anaesthesia to the panoply of techniques used in intensive care. However, obstetric anaesthetists face new challenges – not least, for example, from the rapidly growing cohort of women with surgically ameliorated congenital heart disease. The latter group now represents almost 1% of all pregnant women, and together with the frequent acquired lesions seen in the growing number of refugees, death associated with cardiac disease in pregnancy has become one of the major contributors to maternal mortality in the UK. Moreover, the numbers of such deaths have doubled over the last 15 years. There is never any place for complacency – every maternal death should be considered one too many. So this book is essential reading for every obstetric anaesthetist, and obstetricians would also benefit greatly from carefully studying the lessons that it contains.

Professor Philip Steer BSc MB BS MD FRCOG
Professor of Obstetrics, Faculty of Medicine
Imperial College London
Honorary Consultant Obstetrician, Chelsea and Westminster Hospital
March 2007

Preface

Those who do not remember the past are condemned to repeat it.

George Santayana (1863–1952)

For more than 50 years the Confidential Enquiries into Maternal Deaths in the UK have collected together invaluable information about why mothers die in pregnancy and childbirth. Analysis of the reasons behind the deaths, suggested protocols for avoidance of death in similar cases, and an often sympathetic view of the difficulties facing both mothers and healthcare professionals have led to each triennial publication being essential reading for anyone involved in obstetrics and perinatal medicine.

Often, however, it seemed that the new lessons were eagerly learned, and the old ones quickly forgotten.

For the first time ever, this unique book collects together all of the valuable lessons from recent triennia into one volume. Experts in their fields provide a physiological, pharmacological and evidence-based commentary on the events of each death.

The overall result pays homage to the value of collecting together lessons from the past, and we hope that it will help people to avoid repetition of these situations in the future.

We must thank the Confidential Enquiries into Maternal and Child Health (CEMACH), past and present, for their invaluable cooperation and wholehearted support in the writing of this book, particularly the Chief Executive, Richard Congdon.

Thanks also go to our fellow authors, who have contributed magnificently in such a timely fashion, and finally to our publishers, Radcliffe Publishing, in Oxford, who have turned this important idea into a reality.

Daryl Dob
Griselda Cooper
Anita Holdcroft
March 2007

About the editors

Dr Daryl Dob is a consultant obstetric anaesthetist at Chelsea and Westminster Hospital, London. He has studied, practised and taught obstetric anaesthesia for many years. He is married to Lorraine, and has a daughter, Isis.

Dr Griselda Cooper is a Senior Lecturer in Anaesthesia at the University of Birmingham, and is an honorary consultant anaesthetist at Birmingham Women's Hospital, the University Hospital Birmingham and Birmingham Children's Hospital. She was previously Senior Lecturer at the University of Bristol and a consultant anaesthetist in Dunedin, New Zealand. Her main clinical and research interests are in obstetric anaesthesia and analgesia, areas in which she has published widely. She is a central assessor in anaesthesia for the Confidential Enquiries into Maternal Deaths, and is a Board and Consortium member of the Confidential Enquiries into Maternal and Child Health (CEMACH). She has been a Council member of the Royal College of Anaesthetists (RCA) since 1998, and is currently one of their Vice-Presidents. She has represented the RCA on several Royal College of Obstetrics and Gynaecology (RCOG) and Department of Health working parties related to maternity care. In 2006, she was awarded an OBE for services to medicine in Birmingham. She is married to Brian, a consultant physician, and they have a daughter, Charlotte.

Dr Anita Holdcroft is an academic anaesthetist working at Imperial College London and Chelsea and Westminster Hospital. She completed her undergraduate training at Sheffield University and then at the Royal Postgraduate Medical School and Hammersmith Hospital, before taking up a Senior Lecturer appointment at Charing Cross Medical School, where she completed her MD (in cardiovascular changes during anaesthesia and analgesia) at the West London Hospital. She was appointed Professor of Anaesthesia to the University of Jos, Nigeria and established a new anaesthetic department there, focused on reducing mortality from eclampsia and haemorrhage. She returned to the UK to lead the obstetric anaesthetic service at the Hammersmith Hospital for many years, until the academic anaesthetic department there was closed in 2000, when she relocated to her present post. Anita is known for her work in pain medicine, especially in relation to women. She has written a textbook entitled *Principles and Practice of Obstetric Anaesthesia* and has edited *Core Topics in Pain*. She is on the Editorial Board of the *International Journal for Obstetric Anesthesia*. In addition, she has served as President of the Section Forum on Maternity and the Newborn of the Royal Society of Medicine, as the Co-Chair of the International Association for the Study of Pain Special Interest Group on Sex, Gender and Pain, and is the Deputy Chair of the Medical Academic Staff Committee of the British Medical Association, where she leads developments in women's careers. Anita is the originator and lead of the Obstetric Anaesthetists' Association and the CEMACH Diabetes Project. She has published and presented many papers on obstetric anaesthesia and pain in women, and her expertise is sought internationally through grant-awarding bodies. Her doctoral students are working on the history of obstetric anaesthesia in the UK, especially the role of the Confidential Enquiries into Maternal Deaths, and on the development of new drugs for labour analgesia. She is married to Erasmus, and they have four daughters.

List of contributors

Tom Clutton-Brock MB ChB FRCP FRCA
Senior Lecturer and Head of Department,
Department of Anaesthesia and Intensive Care Medicine,
University of Birmingham, Queen Elizabeth Hospital, Birmingham
Email: T.H.Clutton-Brock@bham.ac.uk

Griselda Cooper OBE FRCA FRCOG
Senior Lecturer in Anaesthesia and Honorary Consultant Anaesthetist,
Birmingham Women's Hospital, Birmingham
Email: gcooper@rcanae.org.uk

Daryl Dob BSc MB BS FRCA
Consultant Anaesthetist, Magill Department of Anaesthesia,
Chelsea and Westminster Hospital, London
Email: Dpdob@aol.com

Michelle Hayes MB BS MD FRCA
Consultant Anaesthetist, Magill Department of Anaesthetics and Intensive Care,
Chelsea and Westminster Hospital, London
Email: michelle.hayes@chelwest.nhs.uk

Anita Holdcroft MB ChB MD FRCA
Reader in Anaesthesia and Consultant (Honorary) Anaesthetist,
Magill Department of Anaesthesia, Imperial College London
and Chelsea and Westminster Hospital, London
Email: a.holdcroft@imperial.ac.uk

Michael Kinsella MB BS FCARCSI
Consultant Obstetric Anaesthetist,
St Michael's Hospital,
United Bristol Healthcare Trust, Bristol
Email: Stephen.Kinsella@ubht.nhs.uk

Mitko Kocarev MD DEEA
Research Fellow, Department of Obstetric Anaesthesia,
St James' University Hospital, Leeds
Email: mkocarev@yahoo.com

Gwyneth Lewis MSc MRCGP FFPH FRCOG
National Clinical Lead for Maternal Health and Maternity Services,
Department of Health, England
Director of the UK Confidential Enquiries into Maternal Deaths on behalf of the
Confidential Enquiries into Maternal and Child Health (CEMACH)
Email: Gwyneth.Lewis@dh.gsi.gov.uk

Gordon Lyons MD FRCA
Consultant Anaesthetist and Director of Obstetric Anaesthesia,
St James' University Hospital, Leeds
Email: glyons@blocked.org.uk

Bernard Norman BSc MB BS FRCA
Consultant Anaesthetist, Magill Department of Anaesthesia,
Chelsea and Westminster Hospital, London
Email: b.norman@lineone.net

Robin Russell MB BS MD FRCA
Consultant Anaesthetist,
Editor, International Journal of Obstetric Anesthesia
Nuffield Department of Anaesthetics, John Radcliffe Hospital, Oxford
Email: robin.russell@nda.ox.ac.uk

Michelle Scott ML BSc MBBS
Specialist Registrar,
Poole General Hospital NHS Trust, Poole
Email: michellescott@doctors.org.uk

Mark Scrutton MB BS FRCA
Consultant Anaesthetist,
St Michael's Hospital, Bristol
Email: m.scrutton@btinternet.com

Mark Stacey MB MChir FRCA
Consultant Obstetric Anaesthetist and Postgraduate Organiser,
Cardiff and Vale NHS Trust, Llandough Hospital, Penarth
Email: airwayman@ntlworld.com

Michael Wee BSc MB ChB FRCA
Lead Consultant Obstetric Anaesthetist,
Poole General Hospital NHS Trust, Poole
Former Hon. Secretary, Obstetric Anaesthetists' Association
and Anaesthetic Assessor for CEMACH, South West Region
Email: m.wee@virgin.net

List of abbreviations

ACE	angiotensin-converting enzyme
AFE	amniotic fluid embolism
APACHE	acute physiology and chronic health evaluation
APTT	activated partial thromboplastin time
ARDS	adult respiratory distress syndrome
BP	blood pressure
BTN	*Beyond the Numbers*
CEMACH	Confidential Enquiries into Maternal and Child Health
CEMD	Confidential Enquiries into Maternal Deaths. Until very recently, the Report has been universally referred to as the UK CEMD. CEMACH, under whose auspices it now falls, has re-titled it as the 'Why Mothers Die Maternal Death Report.' However, for the purposes of this book the old acronym has been retained as it will be more easily recognised by most readers.
CESDI	Confidential Enquiry into Stillbirths and Deaths in Infancy
CMPD	case mix programme database
CNST	Clinical Negligence Scheme for Trusts
COP	colloid oncotic pressure
CRP	C-reactive protein
CSF	cerebrospinal fluid
CT	computerised tomography
CTZ	chemoreceptor trigger zone
CUS	compression ultrasonography
CVC	central venous catheter
CVP	central venous pressure
DGH	district general hospital
DIC	disseminated intravascular coagulation
DISQ	digital impedance signal quantifier
DVT	deep venous thrombosis
ECG	electrocardiogram
ECMO	extracorporeal membrane oxygenation
ERPC	evacuation of retained products of conception
ESR	erythrocyte sedimentation rate

ETT	endotracheal tube
EWS	early warning scoring systems
FFP	fresh frozen plasma
FRC	functional residual capacity
GA	general anaesthesia
GP	general practitioner
HCG	human chorionic gonadotrophin
HDU	high-dependency unit
HELLP	haemolysis, elevated liver enzymes, low platelets
HIV	human immunodeficiency virus
IABP	intra-arterial blood pressure
ICD	International Classification of Diseases, Injuries and Causes of Death
ICNARC	Intensive Care National Audit and Research Centre
ICU	intensive-care unit
IM	intramuscular (in CEMD)
ITU	intensive-therapy unit
LMA	laryngeal mask airway
LMWH	low-molecular-weight heparin
LOS	lower oesophageal sphincter
MEWS	modified early warning scores
MRI	magnetic resonance imaging
MTHFR	5,10-methylenetetrahydrofolate reductase
MW	molecular weight
NIBP	non-invasive blood pressure
NICE	National Institute for Clinical Excellence, now known as National Institute for Health and Clinical Excellence
NNT	number needed to treat
NPSA	National Patient Safety Agency
NSF	National Service Framework
ODA	operating department assistant
ONS	Office for National Statistics
OPCS	Office of Population Censuses and Surveys
PAC	pulmonary artery catheter
PAFC	pulmonary artery flow-directed catheterisation
PARS	patient at risk scores
PCA	patient-controlled analgesia
PCCO	pulse contour cardiac output
PCWP	pulmonary capillary wedge pressure
PE	pulmonary embolism
PPH	postpartum haemorrhage
RCOG	Royal College of Obstetricians and Gynaecologists
RSI	rapid sequence induction
SHO	senior house officer

SpO$_2$	oxygen saturation (in CEMD)
SRDD	Simply RED D-dimer
SVD	spontaneous vaginal delivery
SVR	systemic vascular resistance
TB	tuberculosis
UFH	unfractionated heparin
V/Q	ventilation/perfusion
WBC	white blood count
WHO	World Health Organization

CHAPTER 1

Saving mothers' lives: the contribution of the Confidential Enquiries into Maternal Deaths to improving maternal health in the UK

GWYNETH LEWIS

Whose faces are behind the numbers? What were their stories? What were their dreams? They left behind children and families. They also left behind clues as to why their lives ended so early.[1]

Introduction

This introductory chapter aims to provide a brief background history to the role and impact that the successive Confidential Enquiries into Maternal Deaths (CEMD) have had in helping to improve maternal and newborn health over the past half century in the UK. Their methodology and underlying principles have long been internationally recognised as the 'gold standard' for maternal death reviews and, in modified form, their local application is now helping policy makers and professionals in many resource-poor countries to save more mothers' and newborns' lives.

What's in a name?

The last three Reports in the now 50-year-old triennial series of the CEMD have been entitled *Why Mothers Die*. The introduction of the new title and revised format, first seen in the 1994–96 Report,[2] was intended to revitalise, refocus and re-emphasise the importance of the Enquiry during a period when, to the casual observer, the overall UK maternal mortality rates seemed to have levelled off, or even to have reached an irreducible minimum. This change certainly achieved the intended effect in that the Enquiry once again became required reading for all maternity healthcare professionals, managers, commissioners and policy makers.

Reprints were common, it became a regular bestseller in medical and midwifery circles, and its recommendations once again played a more central role in maternity practice, service and guideline development, audit and policy change.

However, it may be time to move on, and to turn a passive title into an active one, a negative title into a positive one. For although there will always be much to learn, and to question, we should also be celebrating the successes that this Enquiry has achieved over the past 50 years. Undoubtedly, the implementation of its recommendations has saved many lives in the past and, it is hoped, will continue to do so for many years to come.

Therefore changing the title of the Report to something similar to *Why Mothers Survive*, the title of this book, would be a step in the right direction. Some years ago, our South African colleagues started their own Enquiry, which was modified and adapted to their own circumstances but based on lessons learned from the UK. Instead of using a passive title, they chose to celebrate the impact that their work has already had on reducing maternal mortality in their country by calling their Report *Saving Mothers*.[3] It is this, after all, that all of our Enquiries strive to achieve.

Working together to save mothers' lives

All healthcare professionals who provide maternity and other services for pregnant women in the UK are justifiably proud to be part of a maternal healthcare service that places such importance on these Enquiries. It is because of their sustained commitment and continuing support that the Enquiry is able to continue as the highly respected and powerful force for change and improvement that it is today. Each Report's recommendations are valued, and acted on, by many different people at many different levels. Examples include individual health practitioners, the Royal Colleges and other professional organisations, health authorities, Trust risk and general managers, the Clinical Negligence Scheme for Trusts (CNST), as well as central Government and its affiliated agencies. It thus supports the concept of clinical governance in all of its senses.

Reading the Report or preparing a statement for an individual enquiry also forms part of individual, professional, self-reflective learning. As long ago as 1954, it was recognised that participating in a Confidential Enquiry had a 'powerful secondary effect' in that:

> each participant in these Enquiries, however experienced he or she may be, and whether his or her work is undertaken in a teaching hospital, a local hospital, in the community or the patient's home, must have benefited from their educative effect.[4]

Personal experience is therefore a valuable tool for harnessing beneficial changes in individual practice.

Locally, its recommendations help in protocol development, clinical audit and maternity service design and delivery. Nationally, the recommendations of successive Reports have led to the development of several key clinical guidelines and contributed to significant policy changes. Perhaps there is no better example of this than the fact that many of the recommendations of the most recent CEMD[5] are interwoven in the new maternity service standards set out in the National Service Framework (NSF) for Children, Young People and Maternity Services in England.[6]

More recently, the Enquiry extended its remit into wider public health issues, and its findings and recommendations in this area have played a major part in assisting in the development of other, wider policies to help to reduce health inequalities for the poorest in our society. For example, without this Report it would not be known that, even in the UK in the twenty-first century, our most vulnerable pregnant women face an up to 30-fold higher risk of dying than the more privileged.[5] And, by acting on these findings, this Report also played a major part in redefining the philosophy that now expects each individual woman and her family to be at the heart of maternity services designed to meet their own particular needs, rather than vice versa.

Beyond the UK: beyond the numbers

Although pregnancy and childbirth are not entirely risk free, even in developed countries, elsewhere the story is very different. Each day around 1,600 women and over 5,000 newborn babies die due to complications of pregnancy that healthcare professionals have known how to treat for many years. Overall, more than 6 million newborns and 600,000 women die needlessly each year, and a further 20 million women develop long-term complications. More than 80% of these deaths and disabilities could have been prevented at little or no extra cost, even in resource-poor countries. This scandal represents the largest public health discrepancy in the world, and even though the global community is making efforts to reduce it,[7] the current situation is described as a 'patchwork of progress, stagnation and reversal' in the hard-hitting 2005 Annual Report of the World Health Organization (WHO), *Make Every Mother and Child Count*.[8]

If the poorest countries of the world are to begin to make an impact on reducing their maternal mortality rates by 75% by 2015, as set out in the United Nations Millennium Development Goal 5, they need better information about exactly why, where and which of their mothers are dying. Although the causes are generally the same, the reasons why they occur may be different.[7] The barriers to care that these women face may be different. For example, they may be to do with cultural practice, the status of women, lack of money or transport, lack of local facilities or poor clinical care. So in order to develop country- or locality-based specific safe motherhood strategies they need a more accurate diagnosis of the underlying root causes. And it is here that the CEMD methodology and philosophy are helping to make a change.

The methodology used by the Enquiry goes beyond the scientific. Its philosophy, and that of those who participate in its process, also recognise and respect every death as a person, a woman who died before her time, a mother, a member of a family and of a community. It does not demote these women to mere numbers in statistical tables, as the quote at the start of this chapter demonstrates so well. It goes beyond counting numbers to tell the stories of the women who died, in order to learn lessons that may save the lives of those who follow them. Consequently, its methodology and philosophy have now helped to form part of a new strand in the WHO overall global strategy to make pregnancy safer. A maternal mortality review toolkit and programme, *Beyond the Numbers (BTN)*, has recently been introduced which includes advice and practical steps for choosing and implementing one or more of five possible approaches to maternal death reviews adaptable at any level and in any country.[9] These are facility and community death reviews, CEMDs, near-miss reviews and clinical audit. The programme and the rationale behind it are described in more detail in a recent edition of the *British Medical Bulletin*.[10]

To date, representatives from the Health Ministries and professional organisations in over 60 countries have attended *BTN* planning workshops and have already started or are aiming to start one or more of the methodologies soon. These range from parts of Western Europe to remote countries in Central Asia, such as Kyrgyzstan and Moldova, most of the African nation states, several cities in India and its neighbouring countries, as well as the state of Kerala, and several other countries in the Far East and Central America (WHO, personal communication).

The history of confidential maternal death reviews in the UK: the early years

The early 1900s: a push from the professionals

Although the CEMD started universal coverage in England and Wales in 1952, the concept of reviewing local series of maternal deaths was not new. Indeed, the Enquiry's introduction was built upon a system of smaller, local enquiries initiated by concerned healthcare professionals that were already occurring in parts of the UK, usually feeding their results to the Ministries of Health. And, presciently, as with the last three *Why Mothers Die* Reports, these earliest investigations into the causes of high local maternal mortality rates not only considered avoidable clinical factors, but also looked at the provision of services and the social backgrounds of the women who died, and made pertinent clinical and health and social service recommendations.

The first local review known to have reported to a Ministry of Health related to outbreaks of puerperal sepsis in Aberdeen, but this was soon followed by larger-scale studies starting in the late 1920s and early 1930s.[11] This was a time when it became apparent to local healthcare professionals, and women themselves, that although other health indicators such as infant mortality were improving, there was no similar reduction in maternal deaths. The plateau of the maternal death rate in the nineteenth century is shown in Figure 1.1.

Over time, as commitment improved, these small-scale reviews evolved to wider, but not universal, area health authority systems of confidential enquiries reporting to the Ministry of Health. The implementation of at least some of the recommendations in these early reports played a significant part in reducing the maternal mortality rate over the next two decades.

The 1930s and 1940s, which followed the inception of these smaller-scale enquiries, were characterised by a steady decline in the number of women dying from all the leading causes of maternal death at the time, as shown in Figure 1.2.

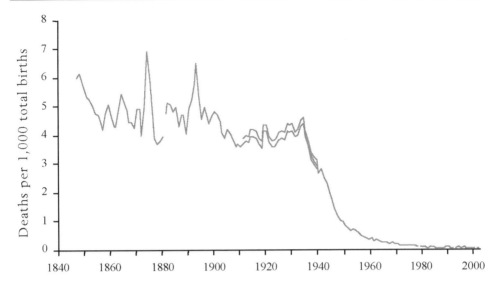

FIGURE 1.1 Maternal mortality expressed as deaths per 1000 births, England and Wales, 1846–2002.[5] Over time the definitions of maternal deaths have changed – hence the broken or in some places overlapping double lines. *Source:* General Register Office, Office of Population Censuses and Surveys and Office for National Statistics mortality statistics.

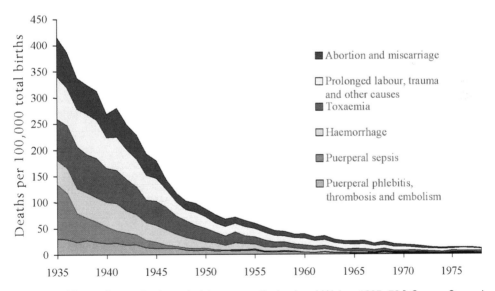

FIGURE 1.2 Maternal mortality by underlying cause, England and Wales, 1935–78.[5] *Source:* General Register Office and Office of Population Censuses and Surveys. Reproduced in *Birth Counts*, Table A10.1.3.

This decline was due in large part to major therapeutic advances, notably prontosil, sulphonamides and penicillin in the case of puerperal deaths from sepsis, and blood transfusions in the case of deaths from haemorrhage. However, the introduction of aseptic techniques as recommended in the early enquiries may have started to reduce mortality from sepsis before the advent of antibiotics, and the constant recommendations to deliver higher-risk women in hospital may have started to reduce deaths from haemorrhage even before the universal introduction of the blood transfusion service. Thus it can be postulated that, even before the introduction of these therapeutic advances, the adoption of the simple and, at the time, non-evidence-based local guidelines may also have played a significant part in the substantial decline in the number of women dying during this period.

However, the reduction in maternal deaths may not have been entirely due to improvements in clinical care. This was also a period of social change and better public health. Access to services also improved as the midwives' role became more widely acknowledged after the 1936 Midwives Act, and general knowledge about the importance of seeking skilled care during pregnancy increased.

Moving to national action

When commenting on the impact of the findings of these earlier enquiries, Sir George Godber, a past Chief Medical Officer for England, stated that 'all this procedure had been intended to do was to secure improvements by the local review of cases, but it was soon apparent that avoidable factors were too often present in antenatal and intranatal care for the opportunity for central remediable action to be ignored'.[12] Thus, in 1952, the Ministry of Health instituted the now ongoing, standardised, national confidential enquiry, which continues to report its findings on a three-yearly basis. At the outset it only covered England and Wales, but as the numbers of maternal deaths declined, its scope was extended in 1985 to include Scotland and Northern Ireland as well.

More detailed historical accounts by Professor Alison McFarlane can be found in the 1997–99 Report[13] and 2002–02 Report, respectively.[5]

The Confidential Enquiry into Maternal Deaths
Aims and objectives

Since its inception, the overall aims and objectives of the Enquiry have remained the same: to save more women's and newborns' lives, to reduce deaths and complications and to improve the quality of maternity services for the benefit of all pregnant women and their families; through the use of guidelines and recommendations, to help ensure that all pregnant and recently delivered women receive the best possible care, delivered in appropriate settings in a way that takes account of, and meets, their individual needs.

The management of the Enquiry

Until quite recently the Enquiry was run by a senior doctor in the women's policy section of the Department of Health for England, in conjunction with colleagues in the other three countries. Placing the management of the Enquiry in the Department of Health enabled policy makers to take account of successive findings and recommendations and use them to help to shape strategic thinking at an early stage. In 2003, the Report merged with the Confidential Enquiry into Stillbirths and Deaths in Infancy (CESDI) to form a new organisation, the Confidential Enquiries into Maternal and Child Health (CEMACH), overall responsibility for which was moved to the National Institute for Clinical Excellence (NICE). In 2005, the responsibility for the Enquiry moved again, to the National Patient Safety Agency (NPSA). Although there is a commitment to publish the next *Why Mothers Die* report, for 2003–2005, at the time of writing the future beyond this is uncertain.

Study methodology

The methodology is best described as an observational study which identifies patterns of practice, service provision and public health issues that may be linked to or affect the reason why certain mothers are more likely to die. This method of reviewing individual deaths has also been described as 'sentinel event reporting', as follows:

> Just as the investigation of an aeroplane accident goes beyond the immediate reasons for the crash to the implications of the design, method of manufacture, maintenance and operation of the plane, so should the study of unnecessary undesirable health events yield crucial information on the scientific, medical, social and personal factors that could lead to better health. Moreover, the evidence collected will not be limited to the factors that yield only to measure of medical control. If there is clear-cut documented evidence that identifiable social, environmental, 'life-style', economic or genetic factors are responsible for special varieties of unnecessary disease, disability, or untimely death, these factors should be identified and eliminated whenever possible.[14]

For the more frequent causes of maternal deaths, the most comprehensive and up-to-date systematic reviews of relevance are produced by the Cochrane Pregnancy and Childbirth Group, the Coordinating Editor of which is a key member of the Enquiry. If a Cochrane Review is of direct relevance to the topics highlighted in the Reports, its evidence is cited to support recommendations. Examples include treatments for eclampsia and pre-eclampsia, and antibiotic prophylaxis before Caesarean section.

However, some causes of maternal death are extremely rare (e.g. Ogilvie's syndrome or cervical pregnancy), and treatment options for these may never have been subjected to formal scientific study. Inevitably, recommendations for avoiding such deaths in the future rely on the best level of evidence available, and sometimes on 'expert opinion.' However, this does not mean that the Report is not evidence based, but merely that, necessarily, the evidence cannot be in the form of a randomised controlled trial or case–control study, due to the relative rarity of the condition.

Another important limitation of more formal trials is that, unless they are very large, they may provide little information about rare but important complications of treatments. Safety issues are therefore sometimes better illuminated by such observational studies than by controlled trials.

The Enquiry process

The basic methodology employed today varies little from that used in the earliest Reports. A complete account of the current process is provided in an Annex to the most recent Report.[5] In summary, each CEMACH Regional Manager, and their other country equivalents, identifies the local cases and initiates the local review process. Deaths are reported by local clinicians, midwives, coroners, pathologists and, increasingly, by other healthcare staff. This information is supplemented by a routine cross-check of death certificates provided by the Office for National Statistics (ONS).

Completed case report forms are assessed locally by assessors in obstetrics, midwifery, pathology, anaesthetics and, newly introduced for 2006, perinatal psychiatry. Once this assessment has been completed, all of the forms are reviewed again by a second tier of national assessors. These assessors, nominated by their respective professional organisations, represent not only the specialties covered by the local assessment, but also public health, obstetric medicine and cardiology, critical care and, as from 2006, general practice and emergency medicine. The final Report is then written by the central assessors in collaboration with their counterparts in all other countries, referring to national experts and the Cochrane database as necessary.

Definitions of maternal mortality

The Enquiry covers the deaths of all women in the UK who died during pregnancy, childbirth or up to 1 year after delivery, or as a result of ectopic pregnancy, termination of pregnancy or fetal loss.

Since 1952, the definition of what constitutes a maternal death has changed in line with successive revisions of the maternal death codes as defined by the International Classification of Diseases, Injuries and Causes of Death (ICD). The early CEMD Reports simply divided maternal deaths into 'true' or 'associated' categories. True deaths were those that today we know as *direct* deaths (i.e. due to obstetric complications and anaesthesia), and the early Reports focused entirely on these, with the addition of cardiac disease, as the effects of rheumatic heart disease were still a major contributor to maternal mortality.

It was not until the introduction of ICD 9 that the major change in terminology was introduced which forms the basis of the current classification system as shown in Table 1.1. This was introduced in the 1982–84 Report.[15] The latest revision, ICD 10, builds on the existing UK practice of including an analysis of *late* deaths (i.e. deaths occurring 43 days or more after delivery). It is hoped that further ICD revisions will again take note of the UK extended case definitions, especially recognising maternal suicide due to puerperal psychosis, a condition uniquely associated with pregnancy, as an *indirect*, or even *direct*, death.

TABLE 1.1 Definitions of maternal deaths

Maternal deaths*	Deaths of women while pregnant or within 42 days of the end of the pregnancy, from any cause related to or aggravated by the pregnancy or its management, but not due to accidental or incidental causes
*Direct**	Deaths resulting from obstetric complications of the pregnant state (pregnancy, labour and puerperium), from interventions, omissions, incorrect treatment, or from a chain of events resulting from any of the above
*Indirect**	Deaths resulting from previous existing disease, or disease that developed during pregnancy and which was not due to direct obstetric causes, but which was aggravated by the physiological effects of pregnancy
Late†	Deaths occurring between 43 days and 1 year after abortion, miscarriage or delivery; they can be due to *direct* or *indirect* causes
Coincidental‡	Deaths from unrelated causes which happen to occur in pregnancy or the puerperium (These deaths often contain important public health information; advice about the correct use of seat belts, and the impact of domestic violence and substance misuse on pregnancy are recent examples)
UK maternal mortality ratio	The number of *direct* and *indirect* deaths per 100,000 live births
UK maternal mortality rate	The number of *direct* and *indirect* deaths per 100,000 deliveries (Deaths due to suicide and hormone-dependent malignancies are included in the numerator, and the denominator includes all deliveries, including still births, after 24 weeks' gestation)

*ICD 9.

†ICD 10.

‡ICD 9 classifies these deaths as 'Fortuitous'.

Guiding principles

From the outset, many key aspects of the CEMD Reports have remained constant, including the following:

- maintaining confidentiality
- ensuring that cases are assessed by recognised and respected healthcare professionals who are expert in their field of practice
- using short case summaries/vignettes as an aid to learning
- identifying and addressing substandard care and remedial actions
- developing clinical guidelines and/or audits
- recommending other actions considered necessary to improve overall maternity service provision
- highlighting new or possible emerging issues, and identifying areas for future research.

Evolving scope and content

The first Reports were very short, containing only a few, albeit major, recommendations. Apart from addressing the biggest causes of maternal mortality at the time, such as haemorrhage, eclampsia, illegal abortion, cardiac disease and anaesthesia, they also focused on issues of service provision, such as the safety of home or nursing home confinements and Caesarean section.[16] As time progressed, the remit of the Reports, and hence the specialties of the professional assessors, expanded to include new areas of clinical concern. In 1982–84, *indirect* causes of death were assessed for the first time, and from 1993 onwards, key aspects relating to wider public health issues. The last three Reports have all included separate chapters, or sections, on issues such as social inequalities and outcomes, access and barriers to care, lifestyle determinants, the impact of domestic violence, and the correct use of seat belts in pregnancy.

Incredible as it now seems, deaths from suicide – the leading cause of maternal death in the UK – were not assessed until the 1994–96 Report.[2] Before this, the numbers had merely been noted as one figure, in one small table, in one short chapter on *fortuitous* deaths. Their subsequent inclusion, and the actions discussed later which took place as a result, vividly demonstrate why going *'beyond the numbers'* is so crucial to the impact of the CEMD Reports and their methodology.

'Avoidable factors' and 'substandard care'

Learning lessons and acting on the results have always been the cornerstone of the enquiry process. The assessors use their judgement as to whether, as first stated in the 1952–54 Report, 'practical and generally accepted standards, attainable under average practice conditions, have been applied, rather than an ideal.'[4] Today's assessors still take a similar view with regard to what might constitute 'reasonable professional practice.'

The term 'substandard care' superseded 'avoidable factors' in the late 1970s, as the latter term was sometimes misinterpreted as meaning that avoiding these factors would have prevented the death. The current term 'substandard care' takes into account not only failures in clinical care but other additional underlying factors which may also have led, even indirectly, to the deaths of these women. These include, for example, failures of inter-disciplinary communication, inappropriate delegation to unsupervised juniors, shortages of staff, lack of access to critical care facilities, lack of blood, staff attitudes and administrative failures in the maternity services.

Ignorant or self-neglectful mothers

It was not until the 1994–96 Report that the attribution of at least some aspects of substandard care to women themselves finally ceased.[2] Since then, the Enquiry and all who contribute to its work have taken the view that if women find it difficult to engage with the services, it is the system which has failed to understand and meet their needs, rather than the fault of the women themselves.

However, even though the earliest Reports frequently tended to blame the women and/or their families, they did recognise that healthcare professionals themselves could do more to engage with the women under their care. As the 1955–57 Report states:

> Nearly one-quarter of potential 'avoidability' in maternal mortality (not including abortions) lies in the patient's refusal or neglect to follow medical advice or to seek such advice. If maternal mortality is to be reduced to the minimum, this factor cannot be dismissed as beyond the influence of the medical and midwifery professions. Some degree of responsibility rests on doctors and midwives to gain the confidence of ignorant or self-neglectful mothers, to study their problems and to help them despite themselves . . . From evidence on the record, in this they [the women] were often supported by relatives in spite of repeated efforts by doctors, midwives and others to persuade them to adopt a more reasonable attitude. Sometimes a woman was undoubtedly influenced by her immediate responsibilities as the mother of her family, and often she was in no fit state to make any decisions at all.[16]

In 2002, the tone was very different:

> Current patterns of antenatal care services are not meeting the needs of the women most at risk of maternal death. Services should be flexible enough to meet the needs of all women, including the vulnerable and hard to reach. The needs of those from the most excluded and less articulate groups in society are of equal if not more importance.[5]

'Telling the Story'

From the outset, every Report has contained anonymous case histories or 'vignettes', either to highlight a specific issue or to make a general point more relevant. Feedback has shown that this unique aspect of the Reports is of utmost importance to individual readers, as well as initiating active teaching sessions for both midwives and doctors. The inclusion of these stories is often cited as the main reason why the reports are so popular and widely read. The following vignette, from the 1958–60 Report, is typical of a vignette of the time:

> A home confinement was arranged for a woman aged 42 expecting her sixth baby. From a purely obstetric point of view, the mechanics of the preceding labours had been reasonably normal. She was known to have 'valvular disease' of her heart, but as the previous labours had been uneventful, both she and her doctor agreed to a home confinement. Later in pregnancy, twins were diagnosed, but even this led to no change in arrangements. As might be expected, this patient experienced extreme tiredness and was 'advised to rest in bed at home', although her circumstances can hardly have been conducive to action on that advice. Labour started prematurely and she died undelivered from acute heart failure.[17]

As time progressed, with the move to hospital-based deliveries, the vignettes tended to become more clinically focused. Many of them still are, but with the additional move towards understanding the wider social determinants of these deaths, some vignettes have been particularly hard hitting. The following case history is taken from the 1997–99 Report:

> A homeless very young teenage primigravida who ran away from home following abuse had an evacuation for retained products of conception. The operation was undertaken by an SHO who perforated the uterus. She appeared to recover from this, and a few weeks later was found in cardiorespiratory arrest suffering from severe hypothermia in a front garden on a freezing cold night. She died shortly after admission to hospital, and at autopsy, although some traces of morphine were found, no specific cause of death was determined. The balance of pathological opinion inclines towards an accidental overdose of morphine, but this could not be accurately proven.
>
> This underage girl, who also clearly was a regular injecting drug user, had at some time been known to social services, but appeared to be out of touch with them at the time of her death. There is no suggestion that any care at all was taken over her future when she was discharged from hospital following the unsatisfactory ERPC. No arrangements appear to have been made to offer her shelter or protection, and after discharge she went to live in the open under a duvet. There was clearly a major failure in the provision of social service support for this vulnerable child, and little attention to her future appears to have been given by the hospital staff.[13]

Saving mothers' lives: the impact of the Enquiries

As time has progressed, it has become clear that the progress of the Enquiry falls into three phases. The early years were mainly characterised by the emphasis on *direct* deaths, ensuring a safe place for delivery and the introduction of the 1967 Abortion Act. The second phase was the era of stronger clinical guideline development and promulgation. The third and current phase is characterised by its extension into psychiatry, inequalities and public health.

The 1950s to the 1970s: from home to hospital and legislative change

Following the introduction of the Enquiries, maternal deaths continued to decline sharply, as shown in Figure 1.3, but then appeared to level off in the mid-1980s. However, although the decline was very real, under-reporting was still an issue in the 1980s and 1990s, particularly in relation to *indirect* deaths.

There were several key aspects to the decline in mortality rates over these first 30 years, which can be grouped roughly as follows:

- the impact of the first recommendations and guidelines
- changes in professional practice and therapeutic advances
- legislation and improvements in public health.

Recommendations and guidelines for place of delivery

A recurring key aspect of the early Reports was the recommendation that better

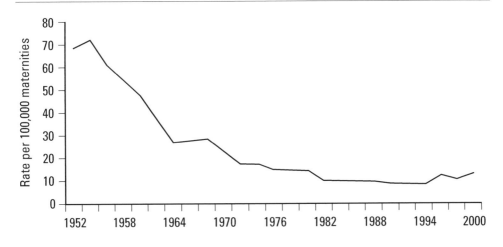

FIGURE 1.3 Maternal deaths for the period 1952–2002. England and Wales data, 1952–84; UK data from 1985 onwards.

selection should take place for women who should be delivered in obstetric units. In 1955–57, eight cases of spontaneous rupture occurred in multiparous women:

> Two were having their eleventh babies, and one each their tenth, ninth, eighth, sixth, fifth and fourth babies. Both the women having their eleventh and tenth babies had been allowed to make arrangements for their confinement to take place at home, surely a most unwise procedure.[16]

The next Report contained the very first set of CEMD guidelines, listing the criteria for women deemed to be suitable for delivery at home or in a GP maternity home.[17] These were as follows.

1 As far as can be ascertained, the woman's general physical state is unimpaired.
2 She is pregnant for the second, third or fourth time, the previous pregnancies, labours and puerperia have been normal, and she is under 35 years of age.
3 She is a primigravida under 30 years of age.
4 She is rhesus positive or is known to have no antibodies.
5 The home conditions are suitable.

These guidelines, and their reiteration in later Reports, must have played a major part in the subsequent changes in service provision. The impact of the move from home or nursing home confinement is demonstrated by the fact that the 1976–78 Report shows only 0.9% of deliveries took place at home, compared with 29% in 1964. In the 1979–81 Report, only four women died at home during delivery, compared with nearly 200 in the 1961–63 triennium.

Therapeutic advances and changes in practice

Deaths from all major obstetric causes decreased significantly during this period. Using anaesthesia and haemorrhage as examples, it is clear that the simple guidelines contained in some of the earlier Reports had a direct impact, resulting in this decline.

The dramatic reduction in the number of maternal deaths due to anaesthesia is one of the major success stories of these earlier Reports, and is discussed in detail in the relevant chapter of the latest Report, and in this book.[5] Regular guidelines, recommendations for advances in practice, education and supervision, and the introduction of new drugs and techniques were all features of these early Reports. As a result, anaesthesia for Caesarean section is now 40 times safer than it was in the 1960s.[5]

The number of deaths due to haemorrhage has similarly declined. In terms of numbers, at least 40 women a year died from haemorrhage in the early 1950s, compared with about three each year more recently. By 1975, the major fall in death rates had occurred, and this improvement is thought to have been partly attributed to the management guidelines which were regularly published in the early Reports, particularly in relation to delivering high-risk women in obstetric units, better clinical management, the presence of an obstetric consultant and the use of flying squads.

Legislation

The early Reports also noted, without comment or recommendations, the devastating numbers of women who died as a result of illegal abortions. This was the leading cause of maternal mortality in the UK until the introduction of the 1967 Abortion Act. However, unsafe abortion is still the leading cause of maternal mortality worldwide.

The first Report described 153 deaths resulting from 'abortion', of which at least 108 had been procured illegally.[4] Around 30 deaths per year due to illegal abortion continued to occur through the rest of the 1950s and the 1960s. Although the first Report was neutral on this issue, the figures themselves had a major effect on the parliamentary debate, and were used to support the introduction of the enabling legislation. During the full first working year of the Abortion Act in 1969, the number of deaths due to illegal abortion fell to 17 and declined thereafter. Several further years passed before there were no deaths due to illegal abortion, demonstrating that legislative changes may take time to deliver benefits in both the availability of services and public awareness.

The 1980s to the mid-1990s: guidelines and indirect deaths

In the mid-1980s the overall mortality rate appeared to plateau, which in some quarters led to a questioning of the need for the Enquiry to continue. However, when the overall rate was broken down into individual *direct* causes of death, as shown in Figure 1.4, subtle but distinct changes in causes of death were noted, which led to concern. This ushered in a new era for the Reports, characterised by more detailed clinical recommendations and guidelines and the inclusion of *indirect* deaths.

The most obvious rise and then sudden decline associated with a specific cause of maternal death in this era of the Report is that due to thromboembolism. The relentless rise in deaths from pulmonary embolism (PE), particularly

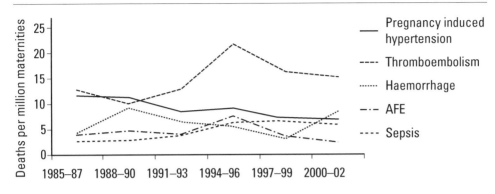

FIGURE 1.4 Trends in direct deaths in the UK, 1985–2002. AFE, Amniotic fluid embolus.

following Caesarean section, which reached its peak in 1994, prompted the Royal College of Obstetricians and Gynaecologists (RCOG) to develop guidelines for thromboprophylaxis during Caesarean section, which were rapidly promulgated throughout the country, and the immediate effects of which can be clearly seen.[18] The more recently found association between deaths from PE and apparently normal vaginal deliveries in obese women has led to further guideline development for the management of this increasingly prevalent group of women.[19]

However, lessons can be forgotten, as the increase in deaths due to haemorrhage around 1985 (*see* Figure 1.4) demonstrates. This led to the need for the guidelines to be reissued, to re-emphasise the need for a consultant obstetrician to be present during the delivery of women with severe placenta praevia, as it was clear that this was no longer happening. However, guidelines will always need constant revision and reiteration, as the following vignette from the 1997–99 Report demonstrates:

> A woman who had suffered a retained placenta with PPH in her previous deliveries (the first being recorded as placenta accreta) had an induced delivery over a weekend with no blood bank on site. When the placenta was retained, there was midwifery delay in calling the [obstetric] registrar. When haemorrhage became profuse there was then a further delay before the registrar called the consultant, and more delay in proceeding to hysterectomy. This was compounded by further delays in obtaining crossmatched blood from a hospital several miles away.[13]

Indirect deaths

As the number of deaths from *direct* obstetric causes continued to decline, the contribution and ascertainment of deaths from *indirect* causes became more significant. In 1994, deaths from *indirect* causes equalled those from *direct* causes, and since then they have steadily risen and, as shown in Figure 1.5, they remain the largest group of maternal deaths overall.

The deaths of women from *indirect* causes are no less important, and the lessons derived from them have led to valuable new recommendations. Apart from deaths due to psychiatric disorders, other examples of *indirect* deaths include those due

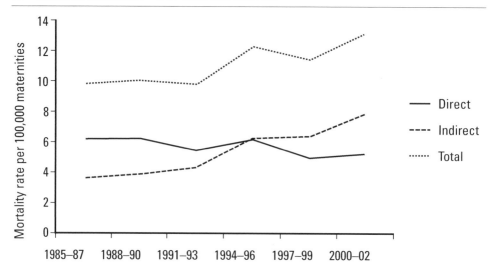

FIGURE 1.5 Direct and indirect mortality rates per 100,000 maternities in the UK, 1985–2002.

to cardiac disease, epilepsy, diabetes, HIV, some cancers and cerebral haemorrhage. Many of these women did not receive appropriate, coordinated, multi-disciplinary care, and these findings in the most recent Report helped to support the development of the NSF standard for local Maternity and Neonatal Care Networks.[5] In the future, women will be able to receive coordinated medical and social care from their specialist physicians, surgeons, psychiatrists or social workers, for example, working together with their maternity colleagues along agreed and shared pathways of care.

1995 onwards: public health and central policy making

The inclusion of public health moved the Report into an era where, perhaps, its influence has never been greater. Apart from highlighting the stark inequalities in outcomes for vulnerable women, it also shows that lifestyle factors result in more women dying. Obesity, smoking, substance misuse and poor overall health are leading to increases in the number of deaths from myocardial infarction, lung cancer and overdoses of recreational drugs. Violence in the home affected many of those who died, some being murdered despite the existence of clear indications for intervention or help. Child protection issues are a new and worrying feature, as is the need for better links with social and other local authority services. Many of these issues are now being addressed through the development of relevant NICE guidelines, the implementation of the NSF, and wider public health initiatives.

Conclusion: unremitting vigilance on a national scale

This chapter has demonstrated how, in a variety of different ways, these Enquiries have played a significant role over the years in helping to improve the health and well-being of all mothers and their babies in the UK. With the passage of time, some issues have changed while others, such as follow-up of non-attenders, remain obstinately the same. New themes have emerged and others have receded. Guidelines and recommendations have been developed, re-enforced, refined and reiterated; often to significant effect. Throughout this long period, the Enquiries have retained the support and affection of all who work, or have worked, in the variety of services that provide care and support for the pregnant women and new mothers whom they serve.

However, some ask the following question, as others have before. What is their worth and utility now? As long ago as 1955–57, the Report enquired:

> Two Reports have now been published. Has work and trouble involved in their production been justified? Can we expect a further and substantial reduction in maternal and perinatal mortality? Is it not probable that an irreducible minimum or hard core must be recognised and is not this figure nearly reached? These and similar questions must have been asked many times . . . not without justification.[16]

This chapter demonstrates that the answer is clear. For even though the Report has changed practice, guidelines and audits are routine, and the number of women dying has been greatly reduced, this change is not yet enough. By continuing to bring the wider and deeper underlying root causes of maternal mortality to the fore, policy makers and healthcare professionals have the information that they need to develop or advocate for services and strategies that can not only improve clinical care but also address the inequalities faced by the most vulnerable women in our society today. For example, without recent Reports the following issues would not have been identified.

- Vulnerable and excluded women in the UK are 30 times more likely to die. This statistic is now at the heart of the new vision for individualised flexible maternity services based around the woman and her family's needs.
- Maternal suicide is the leading cause of maternal death. This finding resulted in the development of a women's mental health strategy, accelerated the development of the new subspecialty of perinatal psychiatry, and provided a vision for a perinatal mental health service available to all.
- At least 15% of the pregnant women who died suffered domestic abuse. This helped to lead to a new national strategy for helping these women, and the production of a handbook for all healthcare professionals to assist them in caring for all other patients as well.[20]
- Multi-agency working allows women to slip through the health and social services net. The findings have led to the development of new joint health and social care guidelines for the coordinated multi-agency management of vulnerable women with socially complex pregnancies, including substance misuse.

The future holds many new challenges. Morbid obesity, HIV, tuberculosis and acquired cardiac disease in particular are all increasingly common causes of death. The increase in the number of deaths from haemorrhage in women who have had a previous Caesarean section is worrying, as are the possible psychological effects of undergoing a medical termination of pregnancy alone, at home. The handling of child protection issues is also causing increasing concern, with women committing suicide or concealing their pregnancies and dying as a result. Finally, demographic changes in our population are already presenting new challenges for the care and management of the many diverse groups of women in our society. For example, none of the 10 asylum-seeking women whose deaths were discussed in the last Report had received appropriate antenatal care.

Therefore the conclusion must be the same as it was for the 1955–57 Report:

> There are grounds for belief that childbirth will continue to become ever more safe and that no small part will be played by an unremitting vigilance on a national scale.[16]

CHAPTER 2

General anaesthesia and failure to ventilate

MARK STACEY

Anaesthesia-related deaths are a small proportion of the overall maternal mortality figures, but in many cases are preventable. Airway skills require a high standard of practice, as problems with the airway are urgent and life threatening. General anaesthesia deaths relate to airway disasters, such as failure to intubate, oxygenate and ventilate. A pregnant woman is at higher risk of airway management difficulties than normal.

Respiratory physiology and pregnancy

The incidence of failed intubation is up to 10 times higher in the obstetric population than in a general surgical population of a similar age. Factors that affect this rate include the increasing incidence of obesity in the obstetric population, increased breast size, and an increase in the use of regional techniques for the management of Caesarean section, leading to a reduction in anaesthetists' experience of general anaesthesia. There is concern that an increase in the use of the laryngeal mask airway (LMA) for general anaesthetics outside obstetrics has led to a decrease in the number of tracheal intubation procedures performed, which may further contribute to loss of skills, particularly the ability to perform bag-and-mask oxygenation and difficult intubation.

Factors that increase the likelihood of airway difficulties at intubation and extubation in pregnant patients[1,2] can be summarised briefly as follows.

Oxygen consumption

This is increased to 40% above normal (from 200 ml/min to 280 ml/min), and is mainly due to the demands of the fetoplacental unit and the uterus.

Decreased functional residual capacity (FRC)

There is an approximately 30% decrease in the third trimester when the diaphragm is displaced cephalad by the enlarging uterus. This reduces both the residual volume and the expiratory reserve volume, such that the FRC is greatly reduced (from 2.7 litres to 2 litres). This is more significant in the supine position, and it removes one of the largest stores of oxygen available to the body, making pregnant women very susceptible to hypoxia during anaesthesia.

Respiratory tract mucosal oedema

Upper airway congestion occurs as a result of increasing progesterone levels leading to an increase in total body water. These hormone effects also lead to vascular engorgement of the respiratory tract, particularly the nasal mucosa (leading to nasal stuffiness and nosebleeds) and the larynx (leading to a decrease in the size of the laryngeal opening). Tongue enlargement may also prohibit compression with the laryngoscope, making direct laryngoscopy difficult. Further swelling occurs in pre-eclampsia. Then, if cricoid pressure is applied excessively or inaccurately, a view of the vocal cords is made even more difficult.

Pregnancy-induced weight gain

A normal parturient may gain 20 kg or more in weight. This weight gain not only increases the risk of difficult intubation, but also increases the likelihood of the need for delivery by Caesarean section. Increasing weight and size of the uterus decrease FRC and hence oxygen reserves. During apnoea this leads to more rapid development of hypoxia. The increased feto–maternal metabolic requirements increase maternal oxygen consumption, further decreasing tolerance to hypoxia. Aortocaval compression in the supine position (common in late pregnancy and made worse by obesity) decreases venous return, cardiac output, blood pressure and uterine blood flow. The left lateral tilt used to minimise these physiological factors may also make intubation more awkward.

Management of airway problems

Many detailed airway management algorithms have been published which deal with every potential complication. The Difficult Airway Society[3] has recently provided a set of simplified algorithms, but does not provide guidance for obstetric general anaesthesia. In order to minimise confusion, the use of a simple protocol, in which the only requirement is the competent use of a small number of airway adjuncts, would be preferable.

In order to maximise safety, it is essential that every anaesthetist has a clear plan for airway management. The Caesarean section under general anaesthesia is no exception. Although catastrophic events may be rare, there is no room for complacency, and appropriate strategies must be taught and practised. Not every problem is predictable, but proper preparation and careful practice will go a long way towards reducing failure. Even in the setting of Caesarean section under general anaesthesia there is still scope for teaching airway skills.

The cases listed below have common features, including obesity, refusal to have a regional technique, inadequate experience on the part of the anaesthetist, poor assessment of the patient, poor airway skills, and lack of planning to prevent failures.

Displacement of tracheal tubes
Oesophageal intubation

CASE 1 (1982–1984)[16]

One patient was given a general anaesthetic for elective Caesarean section by an experienced trainee anaesthetist, following the failure of an epidural block. The anaesthetist failed to intubate, and the patient was *in extremis* from hypoxia before the consultant who was called made further attempts. Finally, an attempt at tracheostomy by the consultant also failed, and the patient died within a few minutes. Autopsy showed that this small woman had an abnormally small larynx and trachea, and that the cause of death was simple anoxia.

INTERVENTIONS		PROBLEMS
SURGICAL	ANAESTHETIC	
Elective Caesarean section	Epidural	Failed
	General anaesthesia	Failed to intubate
	Consultant	Further failure to intubate
	Tracheostomy	
	Death due to simple anoxia	Abnormally small larynx

LESSONS

- Failed intubation should not automatically lead to failed oxygenation.
- A range of small tracheal tubes should always be available.

It is wise to spot a failing epidural early and replace it if necessary. In current practice it is likely that the above scenario would have been followed by spinal or combined spinal and epidural anaesthesia, instead of general anaesthesia. In retrospect, a smaller endotracheal tube or abandoning intubation altogether and providing oxygenation by a mask might have averted this catastrophe. Finally, surgical airways (particularly in situations like this) may not be successful, although success may be improved by practice and by the use of dedicated equipment.

CASE 2 (1982–1984)[16]

In another case, an inexperienced anaesthetist was called for an emergency Caesarean section. He passed an endotracheal tube with difficulty and removed it for further intubation attempts only after cardiac arrest had occurred. Different views were held about the primary contributing factors in this case, including a possible allergic reaction to methohexitone or suxamethonium, but to the assessors it seemed to be more typical of an oesophageal intubation which was maintained until it was too late for resuscitation to succeed.

INTERVENTIONS		PROBLEMS
SURGICAL	ANAESTHETIC	
Emergency Caesarean section	General anaesthesia	Difficult passage of ETT
		Probable oesophageal intubation
	Cardiac arrest	Further intubation attempts

LESSONS

- Inexperienced anaesthetists need support.
- Oxygenation is a priority.
- Capnography (unavailable at the time of this death) should detect oesophageal intubation. A backup monitor must be available.
- In the presence of hypoxia, a high index of suspicion must be maintained unless there is clear evidence of correct tube placement.

CASE 3 (1982–1984)[16]

Another woman was conventionally anaesthetised without difficulty, by face mask, for curettage following a suspected incomplete abortion. The anaesthetist passed an endotracheal tube when laparoscopy was proposed for a probable ectopic pregnancy. The story is then vague and confused, but on balance, the best explanation is that the oesophagus was intubated and death occurred as a result of brain damage due to anoxia. It was unfortunate that the tube was not removed when it disrupted an otherwise uneventful anaesthetic.

| INTERVENTIONS | | PROBLEMS |
SURGICAL	ANAESTHETIC	
Curettage following suspected incomplete abortion	Face-mask anaesthesia	No problem
Laparoscopy for ectopic pregnancy	ETT	Oesophageal intubation
		Hypoxia

LESSONS

- Undiagnosed oesophageal intubation led to death.
- Previous face-mask anaesthesia was uneventful.

This woman had an uneventful mask anaesthetic that was compromised by intubation, almost certainly oesophageal. Her life would probably have been saved if the tube had been removed. Although not available at the time of this death, current practice might include using an LMA or ProSeal LMA if intubation was difficult. This would probably have avoided this situation altogether. This case also demonstrates that the problems of intubation are not confined to individuals in advanced pregnancy.

From 1964 to 1982 the number of anaesthesia-related deaths diminished steadily. This reduction is related to a growing awareness that obstetric anaesthesia cannot safely be left to inexperienced anaesthetists. Care in all of the above cases was substandard and, in many cases, the patients who required the most skilled attention were left to inexperienced staff. Tracheal intubation is a fundamental anaesthetic skill, but good training and practice are essential. The inexperienced are more likely to fail to complete tracheal intubation and should therefore have backup plans rehearsed beforehand. Furthermore, the airway should be formally assessed and an appropriate plan followed.

A trained assistant is an essential part of the team, especially when there are problems with airway management. Therefore all obstetric units should have dedicated operating department practitioners or anaesthetic nurses, who are aware of local guidelines and familiar with the equipment available and its location.

CASE 4 (1985–1987)[17]

A woman who had undergone a Caesarean section previously was scheduled for an elective Caesarean section for cephalopelvic disproportion. She was offered an epidural, but chose a general anaesthetic. She was appropriately prepared, and general anaesthesia was administered using a standard technique with muscle relaxants. Although the intubation was difficult, there was a failure to accept that the tube was in the oesophagus until anoxia caused cardiac arrest and the patient died.

| INTERVENTIONS | | PROBLEMS |
SURGICAL	ANAESTHETIC	
Previous Caesarean section	Anaesthetic technique unknown	No problem noted
Elective Caesarean section	General anaesthesia	Refused epidural
		Difficult intubation
		Reluctance to remove tube because of this difficulty
		Failure to accept oesophageal intubation by anaesthetist

LESSON

- If in doubt, take the endotracheal tube out and reoxygenate the patient.

This woman had had a previous uneventful Caesarean section and had declined a regional technique. Her demise was caused by the failure of the anaesthetist to accept that the endotracheal tube was in the oesophagus and not the trachea. The correct position of the endotracheal tube is best confirmed by the consistent presence of a normally shaped capnograph trace. Other methods are confirmatory and applicable in situations where there is some carbon dioxide emitted from the lungs but the trace is abnormal, such as is seen when cardiac arrest has occurred. Although there is a risk of aspiration if a bag/mask/LMA technique is used subsequent to failed intubation, oesophageal intubation will kill quickly and the balance of risk is to remove a misplaced tube. It is tempting to suggest that this patient might have had the benefits of regional anaesthesia explained more carefully, but even in the late 1980s regional anaesthesia was not readily accepted by patients in the UK.

CASE 5 (1985–1987)[17]

The patient, who was obese, had been given ineffective epidural anaesthesia in a previous pregnancy. She was in labour with a breech presentation, and a trial of vaginal delivery under epidural anaesthesia was planned. The epidural gave good pain relief during labour, and the woman progressed to full dilation of the cervix. There was no progress in the second stage, and the obstetrician considered that a Caesarean section was indicated. The epidural had not been topped up for 2 hours, so a total of 30 ml of 0.5% bupivacaine was given in divided doses over 30 minutes. However, this did not provide adequate anaesthesia for Caesarean section. General anaesthesia was induced, the vocal cords were not visualised at laryngoscopy, but intubation of the trachea was thought to have been achieved using a gum elastic bougie as an introducer. It was stated that the registrar anaesthetist had neither a skilled nurse nor an operating department assistant in attendance. Alcuronium 20 mg was given on return of muscle power, but there was no record of the return of spontaneous respiration or of movements of the reservoir bag. Hypoxia developed, the tube was removed and the patient was manually ventilated with a mask. However, cardiac arrest occurred and during the resuscitation the consultant obstetrician arrived and delivered the baby by breech extraction. Death occurred 2 days later in the intensive-care unit (ICU) as a result of the hypoxic episode.

INTERVENTIONS		PROBLEMS
SURGICAL	ANAESTHETIC	
Previous pregnancy	Ineffective epidural	Previous failed epidural
This labour	Effective epidural	Obesity
Caesarean section	Inadequate block	Failed epidural
	General anaesthetic	No skilled assistance Possible oesophageal intubation
	Alcuronium	No return of muscle power
	ETT removed + bag mask	Hypoxia

LESSONS

- Previous medical history is important.
- Seek adequate help.
- In the case of a difficult intubation, consider removal of the ETT and oxygenation.
- Avoid the use of long-acting muscle relaxants if the airway is compromised.

This obese woman had had a previous ineffective epidural for pregnancy. However, during this labour she had an effective epidural that had not been topped up for 2 hours, which implies that the epidural was probably working. As she failed to progress, a Caesarean section was planned, for which there was no particular urgency. The top-up for the epidural did not work, indicating that the catheter had probably fallen out. It is sensible for the anaesthetist to check the position of the catheter before providing a top-up. As this patient was obese, it would now be worth considering a spinal anaesthetic, although at the time this was a less common procedure. Assessment of her airway should have been properly carried out and an appropriate airway plan developed. This general anaesthetic was made more difficult by the absence of skilled help. The patient became hypoxic when further paralysis was provided by alcuronium. Although after the endotracheal tube was removed, oxygenation was successfully provided with a bag and mask, the patient died 2 weeks later. The case is made all the more poignant by the fact that the obstetrician delivered the baby by breech extraction, which implies that the Caesarean section was an unnecessary operation.

CASES 6 TO 8 (2000–2002)[20]

In this triennium, there were two deaths and one *direct late* death that resulted from oesophageal intubation during anaesthesia. In two of the cases, anaesthesia was being given for urgent Caesarean section, and in one case it was for a presumed ruptured ectopic pregnancy. In all cases, SHO-grade trainees, without immediate senior backup, administered the anaesthetics.

In one case, a death from anaesthesia occurred due to inadequate supervision. The anaesthetist, who was new both to the country and to the hospital, had not undergone any assessment of competence, and gave general anaesthesia without direct supervision or the availability of immediate backup. The woman sustained irreversible brain damage.

LESSONS

- Inexperienced anaesthetists should be trained and supervised.
- Capnography must be available.
- Simulators can be used to practise the management of critical incidents.
- Induction and assessment of competency should be carried out before practice on the delivery suite without direct supervision.

The anaesthetist, who was new to the hospital and also to the country, was completely unfamiliar with the location, culture, equipment or other members of the team. This scenario is therefore instructive in emphasising the need for proper induction processes as well as assessment of clinical capabilities. The CEMD 2000–2002 describe an increase in direct airway-associated deaths following a continuous decline over the previous 30 years. The lack of airway-related deaths in 1996–98 may have been due to a combination of luck and an era of better experience, supervision, higher-quality help and practice of drills. A checklist to minimise airway disasters in obstetrics is shown in Table 2.1.

TABLE 2.1   Checklist for Caesarean section under general anaesthesia[8]

EQUIPMENT	DRUGS DRAWN UP	PATIENT
Visual check of circuit	Thiopentone	Left lateral tilt
Exclude significant leak	Suxamethonium x 2	Review assessment (including airway)
Filter in circuit	Ephedrine/phenylephrine	Check premedication given
Face mask	Atropine	Large-bore intravenous cannula
Check vaporiser level		Intravenous fluids running
Check O_2 delivery from machine		Confirm plan with assistant
Check first-choice laryngoscope		Identify cricoid cartilage
Check second-choice laryngoscope		Optimise head position
7.0 mm COTT prepared	Monitoring	Check second anaesthetist's position
Smaller COTT available		Pre-oxygenate (end-tidal $O_2 > 0.9$ kPa)
Cuff syringe	ECG	Theatre staff scrubbed and ready
Tie or tape	Pulse oximeter	Obstetrician scrubbed and ready
Bougie	NIBP	Paediatrician present
Guedel airway	Capnography	
LMA	(+ second test for tube position)	
Suction working and under pillow		
Stethoscope		
Difficult intubation equipment available		

COTT, cuffed orotracheal tube; LMA, laryngeal mask airway; NIBP, non-invasive blood pressure.

Endobronchial intubation

CASE 9 (1988–1990)[18]

The patient required an emergency planned Caesarean section for pre-eclampsia. During a previous Caesarean section for the same indication, the anaesthetist had noted that the 'inflation pressure was high, suggesting pulmonary oedema.' On this occasion, the anaesthetist (an SHO with 10 months' experience) attempted to give a spinal anaesthetic, but this was abandoned at the patient's request. Anaesthesia was induced with thiopentone and suxamethonium after pre-oxygenation and the application of cricoid pressure, but the trachea could not be intubated. The anaesthetist followed the correct failed intubation procedure until a consultant arrived and intubated the trachea. No gastric contents were visible in the pharynx, and the pulse oximeter readings were normal thoughout the period of manual ventilation and intubation. A few minutes after delivery of the baby, the anaesthetists noted that increased airway pressures were required and that there was an expiratory wheeze. The arterial saturation decreased to 30% and bradycardia developed. The situation failed to respond to repositioning of the tube, or to repeated injections of aminophylline and hydrocortisone. Cardiac arrest occurred, external cardiac compression was started and adrenaline was given. The tube cuff was then deflated and the tube moved down into the trachea and back again. This resulted in a great improvement in ventilation and the restoration of a normal cardiac rhythm. The patient was transferred to the intensive-care unit, where fibre-optic bronchoscopy confirmed that the tube tended to enter the right main bronchus.

The patient was weaned from the ventilator but had diffuse brain damage. After 4 weeks the patient ceased to tolerate the nasotracheal tube, and it was agreed that a tracheostomy should be performed under general anaesthesia. This was initially uneventful, but inflation of the lungs through the tracheostomy tube proved impossible, and the arterial saturation fell to 85%. Fibre-optic bronchoscopy revealed that the tube needed to be withdrawn 5 cm in order to ensure that the tip did not enter the bronchus, but in this position there was too little tube in the trachea for safety. The tracheostomy tube was therefore removed and a tracheal tube was inserted. At this point asystole developed, which failed to respond to treatment.

| INTERVENTIONS | | PROBLEMS |
SURGICAL	ANAESTHETIC	
Previous Caesarean section	General anaesthetic	High inflation pressures
Present Caesarean section	General anaesthetic	Failed spinal anaesthetic
		Lack of experience
		No senior help
		No consideration of previous medical history
		Failed intubation
	Failed intubation drill	
Baby delivered	Wheeze + increasing airway pressure	?Endobronchial intubation
		?Bronchospasm
	Cardiac arrest, epinephrine ETT manoeuvres	
ICU		Fibre-optic bronchoscopy confirms ETT in right main bronchus
After 4 weeks, surgical tracheostomy	Inflation through tracheostomy tube impossible	Very short trachea

---

LESSONS

- A history of difficulty with anaesthetics must be an alert even in the ICU.
- Failures have a compound effect.

This woman had a series of problems. Even when she was improving in the ICU there was no planned care for failure of airway maintenance during the tracheostomy.

CASE 10 (1991–1993)[19]

This woman was of high parity, short and obese. Her consultant obstetrician recommended Caesarean section because of an unstable lie and a history of previous Caesarean section. The anaesthetist was an experienced consultant. The woman was offered regional anaesthesia, but expressed a strong preference for general anaesthesia. Routine preparation took place beforehand. No nasogastric tube was passed.

Induction occurred in the anaesthetic room with no apparent monitoring. An 8.0 mm Oxford endotracheal tube was passed with the aid of a bougie.

The anaesthetist was sure that the tube was correctly placed in the trachea, but hand ventilation proved difficult. The pulse was satisfactory but there was hypotension, although there was no anaphylactic rash. Air entry could not be heard on auscultation. The inspired gas was changed to 100% oxygen with halothane. Ventilation became more and more difficult and the patient became cyanosed. The anaesthetist again considered a misplaced endotracheal tube and checked its position. With the aid of a bougie, the endotracheal tube was replaced with another Oxford tube, but there was no improvement in ventilation and although the pulse was still strong, the pupils were dilating.

The anaesthetist checked the equipment and treated this as a case of anaphylaxis, with intravenous adrenaline and hand ventilation. The ODA went into theatre to fetch the monitoring trolley, and aminophylline and hydrocortisone were given over the next few minutes. An accurate blood pressure could not be recorded. The SaO_2 read 60% when first recorded, but it fell to 40% within 2 minutes. Assistance was summoned and a further dose of suxamethonium was given. The endotracheal tube was changed to a Magill tube without benefit. Caesarean section was performed. Hand ventilation was continued. Atropine and isoprenaline were required for bradycardia. After 10 minutes of hypoxia the consultant anaesthetist called an end to the resuscitation. The anaesthetic registrar arrived and confirmed the position of the tracheal tube through the larynx, and the impossibility of ventilation.

Autopsy revealed haemorrhage into both lungs and collapse of the right lung with pneumothorax on that side. Histology of both lungs and kidneys showed fibrin aggregation which the pathologist considered supported a diagnosis of aggregate anaphylaxis. The problem with the right lung was believed to be secondary to resuscitation. The endotracheal tube was seen extending beyond the carina into the right main bronchus.

INTERVENTIONS		PROBLEMS
SURGICAL	ANAESTHETIC	
Previous Caesarean section	Patient strongly preferred general anaesthesia	Short, obese patient
Scheduled Caesarean section for unstable lie, high parity	Consultant anaesthetist	
	ETT passed with bougie	Ventilation difficult
	Cyanosis	Hypotension No air entry
	ETT changed	?Anaphylaxis
	Cardiac arrest	Collapsed right lung Pneumothorax Anaphylaxis

LESSONS

- Always confirm the position of the endotracheal tube.
- If anaphylaxis is suspected, treat aggressively with adrenaline (epinephrine), but remember that airway obstruction may mimic its presentation.
- Tension pneumothorax must not be forgotten as a differential diagnosis.
- Resuscitation in cardiac arrest includes early Caesarean section.

It is important to use several methods of ensuring accurate placement of an endotracheal tube. Although the capnograph is considered to be the gold standard of accurate endotracheal tube placement, this device may fail – for example, due to a power failure or when stomach contents block the capnograph line. If this case was due to anaphylaxis, early and aggressive use of adrenaline (epinephrine) would be appropriate.

Cardiac arrest may have been due to hypoxia (due to a misplaced endotracheal tube), anaphylaxis, or endobronchial intubation leading to lung collapse. When inserting the endotracheal tube, aim to put the vocal cords at the black line of the tube, and confirm bilateral lung inflation with a stethoscope.

Tracheal tube obstruction

CASES 11 AND 12 (1982–1984)[16]

One patient died undelivered during anaesthesia for elective Caesarean section, as a result of an overinflated cuff which obstructed the lumen of the endotracheal tube. The patient died of anoxia.

In the second case, an endotracheal tube became kinked in the pharynx and obstructed when the patient, who was being anaesthetised for a therapeutic abortion and sterilisation, was left in the care of an operating department assistant. The East Radcliffe ventilator also became disconnected from the fresh gas supply, although this was secondary in importance to the obstruction of the tube. The patient died a few days later from the effects of cerebral anoxia.

| INTERVENTIONS | | PROBLEMS |
SURGICAL	ANAESTHETIC	
Elective Caesarean section Post-delivery sterilisation	General anaesthesia	Anoxia
		Obstructed endotracheal tube
		Ventilator disconnection

LESSONS

- Always check for endotracheal tube obstruction.
- Monitor for disconnection.
- Continual presence of the anaesthetist is mandatory.

Following a rapid-sequence induction, particularly if intubation has been difficult, cuff inflation may be more vigorous than intended. Furthermore, one woman died undelivered. Peri-mortem Caesarean section is an essential part of resuscitation of the parturient who has suffered a cardiac arrest. In the second case, involving a kinked endotracheal tube, passage of a suction catheter or replacement of the tube would have resolved this problem.

CASE 13 (1982–1984)[16]

Another patient died on the operating table due to difficulty with endotracheal intubation. She was undergoing general anaesthesia for an emergency Caesarean section. The registrar anaesthetist could not intubate the patient, who was obese, with a short neck and a small larynx, which could not be seen on laryngoscopy. Once the effect of suxamethonium had worn off, a tracheostomy was attempted, but an airway could not be maintained. This caused haemorrhage into the trachea and lungs, which rapidly filled with blood, and despite help from a consultant who was available within a few minutes, all attempts at resuscitation failed and the patient died undelivered.

	INTERVENTIONS	PROBLEMS
SURGICAL	ANAESTHETIC	
Emergency Caesarean section	General anaesthesia	Short neck, obese patient
		Small larynx not seen
	Effects of suxamethonium wear off	Airway not maintained
	Attempted tracheostomy	Difficult due to short neck and abnormal larynx
		Haemorrhage into lungs

LESSONS

- Difficult intubation is predictable because of the patient's obesity and short neck.
- Good communication with obstetricians and review in an anaesthetic antenatal clinic would have allowed an antenatal plan to be drawn up (e.g. availability of senior help, appropriate fibre-optic equipment and use of a regional technique early in labour).
- Once intubation had failed, oxygenation should have been the priority.
- A practised difficult intubation drill (see Figure 2.1) should be followed.
- A surgical airway is also likely to be difficult to maintain in a patient who has other predictors of difficult intubation.

CASE 14 (1985–1987)[17]

A woman was admitted in labour with a concealed pregnancy. The diastolic pressure was 110 mmHg, and no fetal heartbeat was heard. She received hydralazine intravenously and was delivered of a stillborn infant. The placenta was retained. General anaesthesia, which included thiopentone, suxamethonium, alfentanil and vecuronium, was administered by a junior anaesthetist. The patient failed to breathe postoperatively, and suxamethonium sensitivity was suspected. She was transferred to a high-dependency unit for mechanical ventilation, but 15 minutes later high inflation pressures were recorded and it was considered that her tracheal tube had become obstructed, probably by kinking. Hypoventilation resulted in irreversible brain damage before the tube was inspected and changed. The patient did not regain consciousness, and she died 1 week later. Autopsy revealed pulmonary hypertensive disease, but death was considered to be due to hypoxia secondary to an obstructed endotracheal tube.

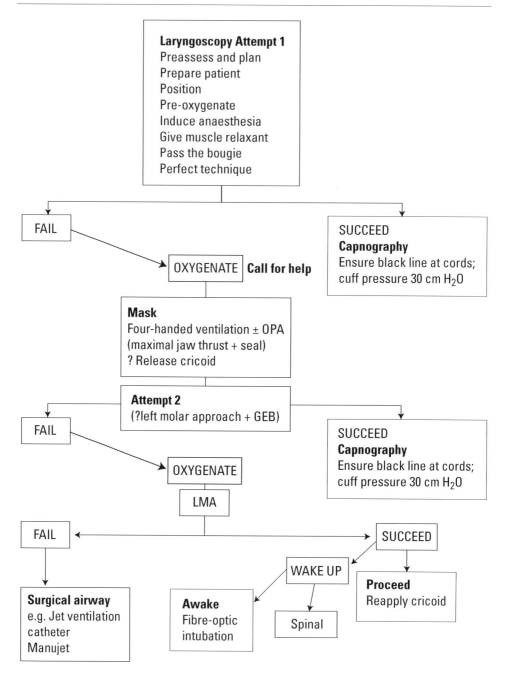

FIGURE 2.1 Failed intubation in obstetrics. Four-handed ventilation describes one anaesthetist providing jaw thrust and holding the mask on with two hands, while the other anaesthetist squeezes the bag with two hands. OPA, oropharyngeal airway; GEB, gum elastic bougie; LMA, laryngeal mask airway.

| INTERVENTIONS | | PROBLEMS |
SURGICAL	ANAESTHETIC	
Removal of retained products of conception	General anaesthetic	Hypertension Stillborn infant Inexperienced anaesthetist
Postoperative	Transferred to HDU for ventilation	Possible suxamethonium sensitivity
	Hypoventilation	High inflation pressures ETT kinked Delays in diagnosis

LESSONS

- High inflation pressures are caused by patient or equipment factors. First disconnect the patient from the machine and check the endotracheal tube patency to assess whether the high airway pressures are due to a machine, breathing system or patient problem. Blocked breathing filters and airway connectors can cause obstruction.
- Patient transfer requires adequate monitoring.

This woman was hypertensive and unwell when she presented in labour and was given a general anaesthetic by a junior anaesthetist for removal of retained products of conception. She failed to breathe postoperatively, and this was attributed to suxamethonium sensitivity. She was then transferred appropriately to the high-dependency unit, but high inflation pressures led to hypoventilation. Presumably the high inflation pressures were thought to be due to patient factors, whereas in fact they were probably due to a kinked tube. This is an example of a confirmatory bias heuristic. Confirmatory bias is the tendency to look for, notice and remember information that fits with our pre-existing expectations.[4] Similarly, information that contradicts such expectations may be ignored or dismissed as unimportant. A plan is persistently followed, even though it is erroneous.

If faced with high inflation pressures, first disconnect the patient from the circuit, use a self-inflating bag to check the patient, and pass a suction catheter down the endotracheal tube to check its patency.[5,6]

Thinking beyond the numbers, this case illustrates the tragedy of loss of lives of both mother and baby, perhaps in a young girl who had not even told her family that she was pregnant.

Patient factors

CASE 15 (1988–1990)[18]

A very obese woman, who smoked 20 cigarettes a day, had chronic hypertension which was well controlled by atenolol. On admission the haemoglobin level was 10.5 g/dl, the blood pressure was 180/90 mmHg and the patient was dyspnoeic at rest. She received a Syntocinon infusion but had a prolonged first stage and was given epidural analgesia by request. Eight hours later it was decided that she should be delivered by Caesarean section. An experienced registrar was called and asked to give a general anaesthetic, since the patient refused to have the operation under an epidural, even though this was working satisfactorily. General anaesthesia was uneventful, a dose of 20 mg of papaveretum having been given intravenously after delivery of the baby. About 15 minutes after the patient had been extubated, the midwife noted that she was cyanosed with laboured breathing, and that the blood pressure was 70/30 mmHg and the pulse rate was 100 beats/min. The anaesthetist was called, gave an intravenous dose of naloxone and then left. Twenty minutes later cardiac arrest occurred. The heart was restarted and the patient was transferred to the intensive-therapy unit, where she died 5 days later without recovering consciousness.

| | INTERVENTIONS | | PROBLEMS |
SURGICAL	ANAESTHETIC		
Labour	Epidural		Smoker
			Very obese
			Hypertensive
Caesarean section	Uneventful general anaesthetic		Refused epidural
	Extubated		
	Recovery		Hypoxic, tachycardic, hypotensive
	Naloxone		Inappropriate

LESSONS

- Obesity is a recognised hazard.
- Consultant input into management decisions concerning refusal of regional techniques is necessary.

■ Appropriate assessment and management of postoperative recovery are essential.

Morbidly obese patients have a high morbidity and mortality, and they are more likely to develop postoperative difficulties after general anaesthesia. Postoperatively such patients should be monitored in a high-dependency unit. This woman became hypoxic, tachycardic and hypotensive (which may have been due to bleeding or obstructive sleep apnoea rather than excess opioids), but was treated with naloxone. When anaesthetists are alerted to postoperative problems, the latter should be followed up rather than assuming that all will be well.

Communication difficulties

CASE 16 (1991–1993)[19]

This patient was an immigrant who underwent Caesarean section. Her husband acted as her interpreter. She refused to give permission for the procedure to be performed under the existing successful epidural block. The anaesthetist was a registrar who received skilled assistance from an operating department assistant and informed the consultant on call.

In addition to oedema due to pre-eclampsia, the patient was obese, with mouth opening limited to two fingers. She was therefore at high risk for general anaesthesia. There was no difficulty with the anaesthetic. She developed post-extubation obstruction of the airway, and attempted re-intubation failed. Neither the vocal cords nor the epiglottis could be seen. Some respiratory effort was occurring, and two attempts were made to insert a laryngeal mask airway (LMA). Suxamethonium was given, and repeated attempts at re-intubation were made with a variety of endotracheal tubes, stylets and bougies. Ventilation via the LMA was also to no avail. A mini-tracheostomy was performed 5 minutes after extubation, but the neck was oedematous and a second attempt was required. Following this there was a rise in SaO_2 (arterial oxygen saturation) of 90%. Bilateral air entry was recorded and some carbon dioxide registered on the capnograph. Slight surgical emphysema developed, and despite further attempts to improve air entry, adrenaline and external cardiac massage were needed. The patient was re-intubated with difficulty by the consultant anaesthetist. However, oxygen saturation remained at 70–80%, and end-tidal CO_2 was less than 0.3 kPa. Bradycardia was resistant to inotropic agents and resuscitation was discontinued.

The autopsy revealed collapsed lungs with no evidence of aspiration of stomach contents. There was mild cutaneous emphysema but, remarkably, no evidence of a tracheostomy entry site into the larynx or trachea. Death was attributed to cerebral hypoxia due to airway obstruction after Caesarean section.

| | INTERVENTIONS | PROBLEMS |
SURGICAL	ANAESTHETIC	
Pre labour	General anaesthesia by registrar	Poor communication
		Patient refused regional anaesthetic
	Skilled assistance	Obesity
		Pre-eclampsia
Caesarean section	Anaesthetic and surgery uneventful	
Post Caesarean section	Extubated	Post-extubation obstruction
	Hypoxia	
	Death	Failed intubation
		Failed oxygenation
		Failed LMA
		Failed surgical airway

LESSONS

- Extubation is as dangerous as intubation.
- Adequate reversal of neuromuscular blocking drugs must be checked with monitors (nerve stimulators and measures of ventilation) prior to extubation.
- An LMA may not be helpful in a scenario of failed intubation and failed oxygenation.
- Surgical airway insertion is a skill that needs practice. It is also likely to be difficult in a patient who is difficult to intubate.
- Simulators may be useful for practising rarely used skills and for training doctors to deal with rarely encountered medical problems.

This case demonstrates the potential difficulty of poor communication through an interpreter leading to the patient refusing to have a regional technique. Initial anaesthesia was uneventful and the problems started after intubation, when a previous intubation risk became a failed intubation. This is another example of obesity predisposing to problems with anaesthesia.

It is also possible that the patient had a tension pneumothorax as a result of the inaccurately placed mini-tracheostomy, which might explain the persistent hypoxia. At the time of this death, experience of LMA use was limited.

CASE 17 (1991–1993)[19]

This patient was obese. Emergency Caesarean section was performed because of failure to progress in labour. The patient refused epidural analgesia. Her general anaesthetic was given by a sub-consultant-grade anaesthetist. Intubation was not difficult, but at surgery her blood was noted to be dark. A low SpO_2 had been noted during the pre-oxygenation, and it fell to 75–80% shortly after induction. Aminophylline was given intra-operatively. There was a typical capnograph trace with end-tidal CO_2 30 mmHg. Airway pressure was high and the patient required 100% oxygen throughout. The endotracheal tube was changed once. There was no evidence of inhalation of gastric contents. The patient could not be extubated until 1 hour after delivery, and was then transferred to the recovery room, where she developed stridor that required reintubation. She then had a cardiac arrest (ventricular fibrillation), was resuscitated and was transferred to the HDU for controlled ventilation. The consultant anaesthetist was not informed until resuscitation was under way. In the HDU the patient developed multiple organ failure, including clinically assessed cerebral anoxia. She died 10 days after delivery after a diagnosis of brainstem death.

INTERVENTIONS		PROBLEMS
SURGICAL	ANAESTHETIC	
Caesarean section	General anaesthetic	Obese
		Refused regional
	Pre-operative low O_2 saturation	?Lung pathology
	100% oxygen throughout	High airway pressure
		Case not discussed with seniors
	Extubated	Very high oxygen requirement
Postoperative	Stridor, therefore reintubated	Consultant finally informed

LESSONS

- There are good anaesthetic reasons for avoiding general anaesthesia.
- Abnormal pre-operative oxygen saturation warrants an early call for help.
- A further high unexplained oxygen requirement warrants referral to senior colleagues or intensive-care specialists before extubation.

This is another example of an obese patient refusing to have a regional anaesthetic, and dying as a result of a general anaesthetic. Although patients have a right to refuse a particular procedure, they should be adequately informed of the dangers of a general anaesthetic, particularly when they are obese. Despite the delivery of 100% oxygen, hypoxia occurred. This may have been predictable from the low oxygen saturation recorded during pre-oxygenation. However, despite the patient's high oxygen requirement she was extubated, with grave consequences.

Airway assessment

If the patient is thought to be difficult to manage under a general anaesthetic, but refuses to have a regional anaesthetic, then a senior anaesthetist with appropriate skills should be present. The patient should be warned at the earliest opportunity in pregnancy of the likelihood of a general anaesthetic.

It is well known that the tests which are used to assess the airway can produce false-positive results. That is, patients are predicted to be difficult to intubate, but subsequently turn out to be easy to intubate. However, the value of these tests lies in alerting the anaesthetist to a potential problem, which should lead to communication with colleagues and the formation of a management plan. There may be occasions when it is appropriate to perform awake nasendoscopy with a fibrescope as part of the airway assessment. This diagnostic test may be considered part of the plan for an awake intubation.

False-negative results may give a false sense of security. The lack of any abnormality in the airway assessment does not exclude airway problems. In an emergency situation, help should be summoned at the earliest opportunity and options for management sought. Depending on the expected difficulty, a regional technique may need to be strongly encouraged. Those patients who are predicted to be difficult to manage early on in their pregnancy should be counselled at an anaesthetic antenatal clinic, and a management plan constructed. It is sensible to place this, together with the results of the assessment, both in the patient's notes and on the delivery suite.

Assessment of the airway is a basic skill and should always be undertaken even if time is short. Anatomical features that indicate potential difficulties in conventional intubation are as follows:
- small jaw
- short neck
- short mandibulothyroid distance
- receding mandible
- protruding maxillary incisors
- fixed head/neck flexion
- large breasts
- large tongue
- obesity.

Consent

There are numerous examples of patients refusing to have a regional technique who are predicted to be difficult to intubate. If the patient continues to refuse a regional technique, an awake fibre-optic intubation by an experienced anaesthetist should be considered. The anaesthetist must act in the patient's best interests, even if this means delaying the surgery in order to perform the awake intubation. Such decisions are not easy, particularly if the obstetrician is concerned about the state of the fetus. Patients need to be informed about the different procedures (e.g. awake intubation on induction or waking with an endotracheal tube in place).

Pre-oxygenation

There is an increase in oxygen consumption of up to 16% at term, compared with non-pregnant controls. In early labour, oxygen consumption increases by a further 20%.[1,2] A healthy non-pregnant patient will sustain up to 3 minutes of apnoea before desaturating. However, a pregnant woman with her increased oxygen requirement and decreased functional residual capacity will desaturate much faster, particularly if she is obese.

Different methods of pre-oxygenation include high-flow oxygen (> 10 litres flow) for 3 minutes, 4 vital-capacity breaths, or preferably awaiting a fractional end-tidal O_2 concentration of more than 0.9. With the advent of respiratory gas monitoring it is probably more sensible to aim for a fractional end-tidal O_2 concentration of more than 0.9 before inducing anaesthesia.[7] This process will be faster if a tight-fitting mask is used to minimise air entrainment. It is likely that even after adequate pre-oxygenation an anaesthetist will have less than 3 minutes for intubation, should it be difficult. While pre-oxygenation is occurring, standard monitoring should be applied. This will also ensure that the capnograph is working and that the supply tube is not blocked or broken.

Equipment preparation

Appropriate drugs for induction of anaesthesia and muscle relaxation should be available at all times in the obstetric unit. A second ampoule of suxamethonium is kept in case there are problems with the first one, and not to aid further attempts at intubation if the first attempt fails. The choice of volatile anaesthetic is debatable, but the non-irritant nature of sevoflurane may have some advantages if airway problems arise and spontaneous ventilation is chosen. It is useful to have a checklist (*see* Table 2.1)[8] in the form of a laminated card that is kept on the anaesthetic machine. The check should be performed at the beginning of the day and before each anaesthetic.

Positioning the mother and using neuromuscular relaxants

Before induction of anaesthesia, the patient should first be positioned on the operating table in theatre in order to avoid aortocaval occlusion. This is usually in the left lateral tilt position. To aid airway manipulation, the head position should be that described as 'sniffing the morning air' (neck flexed, head extended), ensuring that the mouth can be opened maximally. This allows the laryngoscope to take the shortest route between teeth and larynx.

It is important that the first intubation is the best intubation attempt. In order to ensure this, an adequate dose of induction agent, such as thiopentone (4–7 mg/kg), is followed by 100 mg of suxamethonium (more may be required if the patient is very obese, e.g. 1–1.5 mg/kg). After 30 seconds (and not before, so that the drugs have time to work and the patient does not gag), insert the laryngoscope and intubate the trachea with an endotracheal tube of internal diameter 7 mm. It may be sensible to use the gum elastic bougie for the initial attempt at intubation. Successful intubation is confirmed by capnography and normal bilateral breath sounds. Cuff pressure may be measured with a cuff pressure gauge. This can avoid problems of overinflation leading to obstruction. If necessary, a long blade, a short-handle laryngoscope or a McCoy blade can be used for the first intubation. This will allow experience and expertise to be gained with these pieces of equipment before the need to use them when difficulties arise. The use of adult Magill forceps should also be learned.

Assessing position of the tube

Capnography is the gold standard for confirming tracheal placement of the tube. However, bilateral auscultation of the chest is important to confirm correct positioning of the tube within the trachea, particularly if the tube was not seen passing between the vocal cords. In order to avoid endobronchial intubation, place the black line at the level of the vocal cords. It would be prudent to have a backup test to confirm tracheal intubation, in the event of a failure or malfunction of the capnograph, such as the Wee oesophageal detector or a disposable CO_2 detector. Desaturation, detected by pulse oximetry, can be a relatively late sign of an airway problem.

Problems with airway equipment

Airway problems may present with bronchospasm, wheeze or high airway pressures as illustrated in the CEMD cases above. High airway pressures may be due to patient or equipment factors.

With increasingly complex equipment, the risk of it failing is always present. Tracheal tubes or tubing from the anaesthetic circuit may kink or obstruct anywhere from the fresh gas flow outlet to the patient.

In any situation that presents with high airway pressures and falling arterial oxygen saturation, equipment problems should always be ruled out first. Disconnect the endotracheal tube from the whole breathing system and assess obstruction with a self-inflating bag connected directly to the tube itself. If none is available, some authors recommend blowing down the endotracheal tube. If the obstruction is no longer present, it follows that it must be in the machine or breathing system. If the obstruction is still present, then it is in the tracheal tube or distal to it. This information must be ascertained before deciding that the high airway pressures and falling arterial oxygen saturation are caused by a patient problem.

Problems with tracheal tubes may be summarised using the acronym DOPE.[9]

- **D**isplacement (of the tube from the trachea).
- **O**bstruction (of the tube or circuit).
- **P**atient factors (e.g. bronchospasm, pneumothorax).
- **E**quipment.

The following problems have been described:

- foreign body in ETT/breathing circuit
- twisted tubes
- wheels of the anaesthetic machine compressing the breathing circuit
- herniated cuff of ETT
- blockage of a breathing filter (e.g. by pulmonary oedema) (macroscopically the filter may look normal, but it may be impossible to ventilate through). The anaesthetist may change the circuit and the ETT, but not the filter, continuing to think that the patient is the cause of the problem.[5,6]

Failed intubation

If laryngoscopy fails, the priorities are as follows.

1 Oxygenate the patient.
2 Call for help early.

Oxygenation is most likely to be successful if a two-person, four-handed ventilation technique is used with an oropharyngeal airway. It is important that the jaw thrust is applied to the posterior border of the ramus of the mandible (i.e. as close to the posterior margin of the ear as possible), with the thrust being applied towards the ceiling. This manoeuvre ensures that three primary areas of airway obstruction (tongue, epiglottis and soft palate) are bypassed, allowing oxygenation and ventilation to continue. With adequate jaw thrust and a proper mask seal, oxygenation should be possible in most cases, but cricoid pressure may need to be removed or adjusted to improve the airway. The current recommendation for cricoid pressure is to use a force of 30 N (equivalent to a weight of 3 kg). This can be practised on scales, such as those kept in obstetric theatres for weighing babies. Recent debate has focused on the force applied and its distortion of the airway.[10]

If a second attempt at intubation is considered (although patient care must not be compromised), a 'left molar approach' may be successful where conventional laryngoscopy is not.[11] This is described as inserting the laryngoscope directly down the left side of the mouth to access the larynx. It is thought to improve the view because the tongue does not need to be compressed in order to obtain a view of the larynx. Again this particular technique can and should be practised on an intubation manikin or on elective cases before being used in the emergency situation. If the larynx can be seen but cannot be intubated, a smaller tracheal tube may need to be utilised, perhaps using a bougie or Magill forceps to aid intubation. A second ampoule of suxamethonium is kept in the tray in case the first ampoule is dropped, and not to provide further paralysis.

Airway rescue technique

If the second attempt at laryngoscopy is unsuccessful and oxygenation is still difficult, the insertion of a classic laryngeal mask airway (cLMA) is the next step. It may be necessary to ease the degree of cricoid pressure that is being applied to allow proper positioning of the cLMA. If the cLMA insertion is successful and oxygenation is possible, the safest decision is to wake up the mother. Additional help can then be used to provide anaesthesia (e.g. using either a regional technique or awake fibre-optic intubation).

If surgery has to proceed at this point, oxygenation and anaesthesia can be continued with spontaneous ventilation through the LMA, and cricoid pressure reapplied. It may be worth considering fibre-optic tracheal intubation through the LMA to provide a more secure airway. The volatile agents may have to be used to deepen anaesthesia, and this can lead to a reduced uterine tone with increased bleeding.

The Difficult Airway Society has recommended the intubating LMA (Fastrach LMA) or ProSeal™ LMA (pLMA) as alternatives for failed intubation (although the obstetric situation is exempted from these guidelines). However, both devices are larger than the classic LMA, and many anaesthetists are less likely to have experience in their use. A recent case report by Awan et al.[12] describes the successful use of the pLMA in obstetrics, but also advises against its use by the inexperienced in cases of failed intubation.

It is important to decide on a rescue technique before inducing anaesthesia, as a situation of failed intubation and ventilation is not the time to be making such a decision.

The question of whether to proceed with an urgent case of fetal compromise, without tracheal intubation, or to risk the death of the fetus and allow the mother to wake, is a difficult one. In practice, the primary duty of the anaesthetist is to the mother, and there are two absolute indications to continue with surgery, namely maternal cardiac arrest and life-threatening haemorrhage. This should be stressed, and general anaesthesia only continued in exceptional circumstances by an anaesthetist with adequate expertise in the management of such difficult cases.[13] In a maternal cardiac arrest the uterus must be evacuated if cardiopulmonary resuscitation is to have any chance of success. In massive obstetric haemorrhage, bleeding is unlikely to be controlled until the placenta has separated. In other situations it may be sensible to wake up the patient and consider other methods of anaesthesia.

Failed intubation, failed oxygenation: the surgical airway

A purpose-designed cricothyroidotomy kit or jet ventilation catheter with a jet ventilator can be used to provide a surgical airway. All anaesthetists can be trained to put the equipment together and to jet ventilate a dummy before they are faced with a general anaesthetic to be administered to a patient. In a manikin study, four different surgical airways were assessed and some were found to be more technically reliable than others.[14]

Training and assistance

Training using simulator-based scenarios can be useful for practising failed intubation/ventilation. Any of the cases highlighted above can be used as training tools, allowing skills, knowledge of equipment, flexibility of thinking and teamwork to be taught. In the operating theatre, the skill of managing an airway with a mask and oropharyngeal airway needs a raised profile, and should be practised on non-obstetric patients. Any elective obstetric general anaesthetic should be used as a training opportunity to teach a rapid-sequence induction, so long as there are no concerns about the airway. Appropriate senior colleagues should always be available for training and for more difficult patients. Skilled assistance is part of successful management of general anaesthesia, and must be available at all times. It is important that assistants are also trained in and practise failed and difficult intubation drills with the team.

Extubation and postoperative care

If the patient was difficult to intubate, extreme care should be taken during extubation.

There is debate as to whether extubation should be undertaken in the left lateral position or the upright position. The left lateral position is used by radiologists to encourage reflux, whereas sitting upright allows freer excursion of the diaphragm, which is particularly relevant in the obese patient. If the intra-abdominal pressure is high, it is still possible to regurgitate in the sitting or reclining position.

Laryngeal competence is impaired for some hours after anaesthesia, so aspiration of gastric contents is a risk during recovery. Postoperative care should be given in a high-dependency environment, and midwifery staff should be trained to assess and manage airway obstruction. Once recovered, the patient should be fully informed if there has been an airway problem. It is best to give the patient a letter to keep, which clearly describes the problem and its management. A copy of this should be kept in the notes, and the patient's general practitioner should be informed.

Conclusions

It is noteworthy how often obesity has been a predisposing factor in maternal deaths associated with anaesthesia. Although it is unrealistic to expect weight loss once a

CHAPTER 3

General anaesthesia and acid aspiration

MICHELLE SCOTT AND MICHAEL WEE

General anaesthesia predisposes women to gastric acid aspiration. Prevention and management of aspiration are fundamental in reducing deaths associated with aspiration. The dramatic reduction in cases of aspiration since the initiation of the CEMD reports has been secondary to changes in prophylactic antacid measures and the increased use of regional anaesthesia.

CASE 1 (2000–2002)[1]

An obese woman (BMI > 35 kg/m^2) died after aspiration of gastric contents following failure to intubate the trachea after induction of general anaesthesia for Caesarean section. She had declined a regional block because of needle phobia. The assessors were unable to determine whether the woman had received antacid prophylaxis.

INTERVENTIONS		PROBLEMS
SURGICAL	ANAESTHETIC	
Caesarean section	General anaesthetic	Obesity
		Refusal of regional anaesthesia
		Needle phobia
		Failure to intubate
		Probable lack of antacid prophylaxis

LESSONS

- Obese patients and patients with needle phobia require anaesthetic assessment antenatally, with the formation of a management plan.
- Failed intubation drills should be practised.
- Antacid prophylaxis should be given and documented.

Recognition and incidence of gastric acid aspiration into the lungs

Many investigators have tried to elucidate the true incidence of morbidity and mortality related to aspiration in obstetric anaesthesia. Attempts to clarify the incidence have been hampered by the rare nature of this complication and by incomplete data collection with regard to exact numbers of general anaesthetics for obstetric procedures. Based on the assumption that approximately 24% of births in the UK are by Caesarean section,[2] and secondary to the increase in procedures performed under regional anaesthesia, about 3% of women will require a general anaesthetic and thus be exposed to the risk of aspiration. However, the figures will be higher because general anaesthesia is used for pre- and postpartum procedures.

Curtis Mendelson was the first investigator to ascertain the exact nature of this problem.[3] He retrospectively reviewed case notes of 44,016 pregnancies from 1932 to 1945, and identified 66 cases of aspiration (incidence 0.15%). Further experiments in rabbits showed that the nature, volume and pH of the aspirate were critical in determining the ensuing clinical picture and subsequent pathology. While taking into account the limitations of animal experiments, Mendelson's advice changed obstetric anaesthetic practice. He advocated the following:

- withholding food during labour
- increasing the use of regional anaesthesia
- administration of antacids
- emptying of the stomach prior to general anaesthesia
- competent administration of general anaesthesia.

Subsequently, the CEMD triennial reports have shown a steady decline in the numbers of deaths related to pulmonary aspiration, with 18 deaths in 1964–66, 11 deaths in 1976–78, and 1 death each in 1991–93 and 2000–2002.

It is thought that aspiration may occur in up to 1 in 3,000 anaesthetics of all types.[4] It occurs during induction of or recovery from anaesthesia or any loss of consciousness (pathological or pharmacological) – that is, in all situations where protection of the larynx is breached. 'Silent' aspiration has been implicated in a number of postoperative pulmonary abnormalities. Mortality after aspiration ranges from 3% to 70%. This huge variation is considered to be dependent on the nature of the aspirate and the therapies used. Morbidity is also difficult to ascertain, but can vary from simple bronchospasm and/or mild hypoxia to lung abscesses and myocardial infarction.[5,6]

CASE 2 (1991–1993)[1]

This patient required emergency Caesarean section for fetal distress. The anaesthetist was of sub-consultant grade and skilled help was available. The consultant anaesthetist was not informed because no special abnormalities were recognised pre-operatively. Standard preparation and induction took place, although ranitidine was not given exactly in accordance with the unit protocol. Secretions had been noted in the pharynx before intubation. These secretions were removed by suction and the endotracheal tube was passed initially into the right main bronchus (SpO_2 of 90%). This was corrected and the SpO_2 increased to 97–98%. Thereafter the operation was uneventful except for excess blood loss. Saline and Haemaccel® were administered. Blood was not available during the operation, as the haematologist was involved elsewhere. Uncrossmatched blood was held in the maternity unit but was not given, although the patient was group B positive with no significant antibodies present.

The patient had a period of serious hypotension beginning shortly after induction of anaesthesia. Despite this, she was transferred after delivery to the postnatal ward, where a blood transfusion was commenced. She was visited by the on-call obstetrician, her blood transfusion was speeded up, Syntocinon was given because of a poorly contracted uterus, and oxygen by mask was prescribed but poorly tolerated. Her pulse rate was 160 beats/min, and additional analgesia was given. Antibiotics were started, as it had been noted that the patient had a cough and was drowsy. She had been febrile pre-operatively. Six hours later she was oliguric and hypoxic. Frusemide was given, and it was considered that she had aspirated stomach contents during induction of anaesthesia and/or while hypotensive and obtunded on the postnatal ward. Hydrocortisone was given, and the associate specialist in general medicine was consulted. The patient was transferred to another hospital to receive intensive therapy, and from there she was transferred to a teaching centre for extracorporeal membrane oxygenation for her ARDS. She died 21 days after delivery.

| INTERVENTIONS | | PROBLEMS |
SURGICAL	ANAESTHETIC	
Caesarean section	General anaesthetic	Emergency
		Ranitidine not given as per protocol
		Pharyngeal secretions
		Right main bronchus intubation
		Haemorrhage
		Hypoxia
		Hypotension
		Reduced Glasgow Coma Score

LESSONS

- Antacids should be administered in accordance with guidelines.
- Pharyngeal secretions should arouse suspicion of possible aspiration.
- A reduction in the level of consciousness should generate an alert for antacid prophylaxis and prevention of risk of aspiration, especially in a parturient.
- Obtunded and high-risk patients should receive high-dependency care.
- Tachycardia may be secondary to hypovolaemia or infection.
- The use of steroids is controversial.

CASE 3 (1988–1990)[1]

This patient was obese and smoked over 30 cigarettes per day. She had required a Caesarean section for her first child because of fetal distress and failure to progress, but her second pregnancy had resulted in a normal delivery. The third pregnancy proceeded normally until 34 weeks' gestation, when the patient was found to be anaemic. On the assumption that this was due to an iron deficiency, she was prescribed iron. However, the anaemia was in fact macrocytic. She was admitted at 39 weeks with indigestion and vomiting and treated with ranitidine 150 mg twice daily for 3 days. Labour was then induced, but the head failed to engage and fetal tachycardia developed, so it was decided that the woman should have a Caesarean section under general anaesthesia. She had received ranitidine 50 mg and pethidine 100 mg IM 2 hours before the operation, together with 800 ml of crystalloid solution. The haemoglobin level was 7.8 g/dl. The anaesthetist, who was very experienced, was aware that the intubation had proved difficult at the last operation, and noted that the patient had a short neck and a receding chin. The patient was given 30 ml of sodium citrate orally, placed supine with a left lateral tilt, and pre-oxygenated. Anaesthesia was then induced while cricoid pressure was applied. The larynx could not be visualised with a short blade, but by substituting a long blade the anaesthetist was able to visualise the arytenoid cartilages and to intubate the trachea with the aid of a curved stylet. The patient did not become cyanosed and no gastric contents were observed in the pharynx. Anaesthesia was uneventful. One unit of packed cells was given during the first 20 minutes of the operation, a second unit during the next hour, and a third unit during the next 4 hours. Blood loss was estimated to be 400 ml. At the end of the operation ventilation was inadequate and two doses of atropine and neostigmine were given, although neuromuscular function was not tested with a nerve stimulator. Ventilation was assisted for the next 15 minutes, and the tube was then removed with the patient in the supine position. It was noted that there were profuse pharyngeal secretions, which were removed by means of a nasopharyngeal suction catheter. The patient was transferred to the recovery area and given 30 mg of papaveretum and 12.5 mg of prochlorperazine. Two hours after the end of the operation, when the patient was transferred to the postnatal ward, the midwife noted that she was drowsy, and that she was very 'chesty' and wanted to cough. The blood pressure was 90/50 mmHg, the pulse rate was 94 beats/min and the temperature was 37.4°C. Four hours later the blood pressure was found to be 100/40 mmHg, the pulse rate was 120 beats/min and the respiration rate was 50 breaths/min. The midwife called the obstetric SHO, who noted that the patient was restless and cyanosed. Blood-gas analysis showed that the arterial PO_2 was 5.8 kPa while breathing approximately 40% oxygen. Treatment with frusemide, hydrocortisone, antibiotics and nebulised salbutamol was started, and the patient was transferred to a medical ward for approximately 5 hours. Twelve hours after the end of the operation she was transferred to an intensive-therapy unit, where she died 10 days later from ARDS.

	INTERVENTIONS		PROBLEMS
SURGICAL		ANAESTHETIC	
Admission			Indigestion and vomiting treated with ranitidine
			Cause of nausea and vomiting not elucidated
Caesarean section		General anaesthetic	Pethidine given pre-operatively
			Delay in intubation
Postoperative			Inadequate ventilation
			Pharyngeal secretions on extubation

LESSONS

- High-risk patients require antenatal assessment and a management plan.
- Neuromuscular function should be monitored with a nerve stimulator.
- Pharyngeal secretions should trigger a high index of suspicion of pulmonary aspiration.
- Postoperative monitoring on a high-dependency unit and regular review by experienced staff are indicated.

CASE 4 (1988–1990)[1]

This patient had suffered a *Haemophilus influenzae* chest infection during her last pregnancy, and in her current pregnancy was admitted to hospital at 37 weeks' gestation with a chest infection that was treated with erythromycin. Two days later she required a Caesarean section due to fetal distress. The anaesthetic was administered by an experienced registrar, but he was unable to intubate the trachea. While the anaesthetist was ventilating the patient by face mask the obstetrician found that the cervix was fully dilated, and so delivered the infant per vaginum with forceps. Following delivery the trachea was intubated by a more senior anaesthetist. Although no gastric contents were seen in the pharynx, there was bloodstained fluid in the trachea. At the end of the operation the arterial PO_2 was low and there were bilateral infiltrations in the lung fields, so the patient was transferred to the ITU, where she died 6 days later.

INTERVENTIONS		PROBLEMS
SURGICAL	ANAESTHETIC	
Admission at 37 weeks		*Haemophilus* chest infection
Caesarean section	General anaesthetic	Fetal distress
		Failed intubation by first anaesthetist Ventilated by face mask
Postoperative		Arterial hypoxia

LESSONS

- Compromised by chest infection.
- Regional anaesthesia would have been preferred if there were no contraindications, such as signs of systemic infection.

- Aspiration prophylaxis should be recorded.
- Careful pre-anaesthetic assessment of the patient might have allowed detection of a possible difficult intubation.
- Ventilation by face mask does not protect the airway.

Aspirated material

The material aspirated is potentially one of three types.

- *Particle related*. Particulate matter causes acute airway obstruction, resulting in hypoxia and possible immediate death. Mendelson's study included 5 cases of patients aspirating solid material, 2 of whom died, in his opinion, from suffocation.
- *Acid related*. The concept of critical pH and critical volume of aspirate was introduced by Roberts and Shirley in 1974.[7] After conducting experiments in monkeys, they extrapolated the idea to humans that a pH of 2.5 or less and a volume of greater than 0.4 ml/kg (approximately 25 ml) results in damage to the lungs. At > 1.0 ml/kg, death or severe aspiration occurs. However, no human studies have substantiated this. Mendelson showed that if the acid vomit is neutralised prior to injection into the trachea, the radiological findings of aspiration do not occur. The harmful effects of the acid are caused by immediate direct tissue injury and secondary to the inflammatory response.
- *Bacteria related*. As gastric contents are not sterile, lung infections are relatively common. The organism involved depends on whether the patient has a community-acquired or hospital-acquired infection.

Scientific basis of management

Gastrointestinal tract anatomy and secretion

The parietal cells within the stomach secrete hydrochloric acid (HCl), with a resulting pH of 1–1.5 under normal circumstances. This provides an optimal environment for pepsin activity and protein breakdown. Histamine, acetylcholine and gastrin act upon specific receptors within the parietal-cell basolateral membrane to stimulate acid secretion. Factors such as somatostatin, epidermal growth factor, β-agonists and enteroglucagon inhibit acid secretion, via unknown mechanisms. Stimulation of the receptors within the basolateral membrane leads to the production of secondary messengers, with resulting phosphorylation of intracellular proteins and release of calcium. These secondary messengers ultimately result in the breakdown of water molecules to release H^+ ions. A chloride (Cl^-)/bicarbonate (HCO_3^-) exchanger at the basolateral membrane rapidly moves HCO_3^- into the blood. This flow of HCO_3^- into the blood, known as the 'alkaline tide', counteracts the removal of H^+ from the blood. This is necessary for acid secretion.

The apical cell membrane contains the gastric proton pump (H^+/K^+ ATPase), which actively pumps the H^+ out of the cell in exchange for K^+. Concurrently, the

Cl$^-$/HCO$_3^-$ exchanger pumps Cl$^-$ via the basolateral membrane. These ions then 'leak' into the gastric lumen, down their electrochemical gradient.

Regulation of gastric acid secretion occurs in three phases:

1 cephalic phase – under the influence of the vagus nerve, resulting in release of acetylcholine and inhibition of somatostatin release
2 gastric phase – amino acids and peptides stimulate the parietal cells to release acid; the resulting rise in H$^+$ concentration directly inhibits its further release
3 intestinal phase – the presence of peptides within the intestines and the blood precipitates further acid secretion. However, high levels of fatty acids within the intestines inhibit gastric acid secretion.

Pregnancy is associated with a decrease in the total acid content of the stomach.[8] This hypochlorhydria appears to be associated with a decrease in plasma gastrin levels. In addition, provocation of acid secretion with test meals and histamine appears to be less effective. This effect is maximal at 30 weeks' gestation, and returns to normal levels by term. No studies have elucidated the possible changes in acid levels during labour, as most patients automatically receive antacid prophylaxis.

The anatomical changes associated with the enlarging gravid uterus have little effect on gastrointestinal motility.[9] However, rising levels of progesterone have an inhibitory effect on gastrointestinal motility as measured by intestinal transit time. The effect of pregnancy on gastric emptying has also been widely investigated. Using either paracetamol absorption as an indirect measure of gastric emptying, or ultrasound examination, no demonstrable delay in gastric emptying has been demonstrated during pregnancy.[10–13] During labour, gastric emptying is markedly delayed, an effect that is compounded by the administration of opioid analgesics.

Sphincters

The oesophagus has two sphincters, namely the upper and lower oesophageal sphincters. The upper oesophageal sphincter is composed of muscle from cricopharyngeus and circular smooth muscle. Its normal action is to keep the oesophageal inlet closed with a high resting intraluminal pressure of 50–100 mmHg (6.7–13.3 kPa). The sphincter opens upon swallowing.

The lower oesophageal sphincter (LOS) is the other sphincter protecting the airway from regurgitation of gastric contents. It is a segment of tonically contracted smooth muscle, 3–4 cm long, at the distal end of the oesophagus, below the diaphragm. The LOS must be dynamic in order to prevent reflux in all situations, including swallowing, recumbency and abdominal straining.[17] The oesophagus has two layers of muscle, the inner circular muscle layer acting as a physiological sphincter. LOS action is enhanced by the crural portion of the diaphragm, which forms a pinch-cock mechanism around the distal oesophagus. This diaphragmatic mechanism is especially important during inspiration, when intrathoracic pressure is negative. In addition, the oesophagus enters the stomach at an oblique angle, thus further enhancing the LOS anti-reflux mechanism.

The resting pressure of the LOS is 15–30 mmHg above the intra-gastric pressure.

This varies with posture, breathing, movement and abdominal distension. Control of LOS tone is by both myogenic and neurogenic cholinergic mechanisms. The LOS undergoes brief episodes (< 35 seconds) of relaxation unrelated to swallowing or peristalsis secondary to vagal nerve stimulation. Hormones also influence LOS tone (see Table 3.1). A decrease in LOS tone is seen from early pregnancy. With the onset of swallowing, the LOS starts to relax (under the influence of nitric oxide), with complete relaxation occurring by the time the peristaltic wave and food bolus arrive. Once the food bolus has passed through the LOS, the latter actively contracts to 1–15 mmHg above the resting tone for 10–15 seconds before restoring its normal tonic contraction.

TABLE 3.1 Factors that increase or decrease lower oesophageal sphincter (LOS) pressure

	INCREASE LOS PRESSURE	DECREASE LOS PRESSURE
Hormones	Gastrin, motilin	Secretin, glucagon, gastric intestinal peptide, vasoactive intestinal peptide, progesterone
Neural stimulation	α-Adrenergic agonists, β-adrenergic antagonists, cholinergic agents	α-Adrenergic antagonists, β-adrenergic agonists, cholinergic antagonists, serotonin
Drugs	Metoclopramide, domperidone (cisapride*)	Nitrates, calcium-channel blockers, morphine, diazepam, barbiturates

*Not recommended for use because of adverse reactions.

Regurgitation and vomiting

CASE 5 (1988–1990)[1]

This patient died 45 days after receiving an anaesthetic, and has been classified as a *late* death. She had a prolonged second stage with transverse arrest of the fetal head. Two 100 mg doses of pethidine were given during labour. Since the patient had refused epidural analgesia, it was agreed that a trial of forceps should be undertaken under general anaesthesia. Metoclopramide 10 mg and ranitidine 50 mg were given intramuscularly, and 10 ml of a propretiary antacid were given orally. Anaesthesia was induced 20 minutes later with thiopentone and suxamethonium, with cricoid pressure being applied by a trained assistant. The patient regurgitated a large quantity of gastric contents, and laryngoscopy revealed that some of this material had entered the trachea. Intubation was accomplished easily and the trachea was suctioned, but the inflation pressure remained high despite the intravenous administration of aminophylline and methylprednisolone. The patient was transferred to the ITU but died from a suppurative bronchopneumonia and renal failure.

INTERVENTIONS		PROBLEMS
SURGICAL	ANAESTHETIC	
Admitted in labour		Prolonged second stage
		Pethidine given
		Refused spinal or epidural anaesthesia
Trial of forceps	General anaesthetic	Regurgitation of large amounts of aspirate
		Aspirate seen in trachea
		High ventilation pressures
Postoperative		Suppurative bronchopneumonia

LESSONS

- Parenteral opioids increase gastric stasis.
- Metoclopramide is less effective at gastric emptying if parenteral opioids have already been given.
- Refusal of regional anaesthesia can increase risk, and senior anaesthetic input should be considered.
- 'Proprietary' antacid was inadequate.
- Theoretically, correct application of cricoid pressure should prevent regurgitation of gastric contents into the oropharynx.
- The use of high-dose steroids following aspiration is controversial.

Regurgitation is the passive passage of gastric contents, including acid, from the stomach along the oesophagus into the pharynx. This process is normally prevented by the action of the LOS. Most people experience some degree of gastro-oesophageal reflux into the oesophagus hourly. These episodes normally result in no symptoms. If there is pathological gastro-oesophageal reflux, a range of symptoms can result, ranging from mild heartburn to chronic oesophageal mucosal damage with or without dysphagia/odynophagia. The latter is a sharp substernal pain with swallowing. It may limit oral intake and is caused by oesophageal ulceration, especially with infectious oesophagitis.

Heartburn is reported to occur in approximately 30–50% of all pregnancies.[14–17] Women commonly experience onset of symptoms after 5 months of pregnancy, with cessation of symptoms after delivery. Pregnancy is the commonest cause of gastro-oesophageal reflux disease associated with heartburn, other than oesophagitis. Frequently, recurrence occurs with subsequent pregnancies.

The pathogenesis of gastro-oesophageal reflux in pregnancy is multi-factorial. Causes include the following:
- effects of hormones on the LOS
- increased intra-abdominal pressure

- shortening of the LOS
- delayed gastric emptying
- acid content of the gastric reflux.

The absolute LOS pressure necessary for gastro-oesophageal reflux is less than 6 mmHg. Studies on pregnant women pre- and postpartum have shown that the dose–response curve to acetylcholine and gastrin was blunted by oestrogen and progesterone. Oestrogen alone appears to have no effect, whereas progesterone alters LOS responses. With both oestrogen and progesterone a synergistic effect is seen based on oestrogen acting as a primer. To assess how early these changes in the LOS tone can occur, studies were performed on women before and after termination of pregnancy (with a mean gestation of 16 weeks). It was found that although the LOS pressure was the same both before and after surgery, the women showed a diminished response to protein meals and injection with methacholine prior to surgery. This response demonstrates that hormones influence the LOS function from early pregnancy, and such changes are maintained during pregnancy due to altered hormone levels.

Physical factors increase intra-abdominal pressure. Pressure from the expanding gravid uterus is marked during the last trimester, irrespective of position, but this is exacerbated in the lithotomy and Trendelenberg positions. The result is an increase in the risk of regurgitation during procedures performed in labour. In addition, due to upward displacement of the LOS into the thorax, the negative pressure generated within the thorax may make the LOS less capable of resisting reflux.

Vomiting is the reflex involving retrograde passage of gastric contents through the mouth. This is often preceded by nausea with or without retching. It occurs in 25–55% of pregnant women (compared to 66% of pregnant women suffering from gastro-oesophageal reflux) via hormone-related mechanisms (e.g. elevated β-HCG, progesterone and oestrogen) as well as psychological factors.

The vomiting reflex integrates three processes – the emetic detectors, pathway integration and motor output.[18–20] The emetic detectors are subdivided into mechanoreceptors and chemoreceptors. The mechanoreceptors are located within the gut and are activated by local damage, excess distension or contraction. The chemoreceptors are located within the gut mucosa and detect noxious stimuli. These stimuli are transmitted via the autonomic afferents. The chemoreceptor trigger zone (CTZ), located within the area postrema in the floor of the fourth ventricle, detects bloodborne emetic agents. The blood–brain barrier in this area is poorly developed, thus aiding this function. The CTZ has a high density of dopaminergic (D_2) receptors and serotoninergic (5-HT_3) receptors. Impulses from the CTZ are passed on to the vomiting centre within the medulla, where all afferent information is integrated and processed. Other emetic stimuli bypass the CTZ and are relayed directly to the vomiting centre via the solitary tract nucleus (i.e. the vagus with 5-HT_3, D_2, muscarinic (ACh) and histamine (H) receptors), the cerebellum (which integrates labyrinthine and vestibular input, e.g. morning sickness), higher brainstem and/or cortical structures.

The vomiting centre integrates this afferent input and produces an efferent response, sending out impulses to the respiratory and vasomotor centres within the brainstem. The vagal motor neurons supplying the gut and heart originate in the dorsal motor vagal nucleus and nucleus ambiguus. The dorsal and ventral respiratory centres which regulate the phrenic nerve output are controlled by parasympathetic activity. The vomiting centre also sends out efferents to the cranial nerves (trigeminal, facial, glossopharyngeal and hypoglossal), the nerves to the upper gastrointestinal tract and through the spine to the diaphragm and abdominal muscles.

The efferent motor activity produces the following physiological pattern of vomiting:

1   a pre-ejection phase with visceral effects such as nausea, reduced gastric tone, absent or reduced gastric peristalsis, increased duodenal tone, sweating, pupillary dilatation, salivation, tachycardia and altered breathing patterns
2   an ejection phase during which the breath is held in mid-inspiration, the glottis closes, the abdominal muscles and diaphragm contract, the LOS relaxes and the gastric contents are expelled.

In the awake state the glottis closes before the gastric contents are expelled, in order to prevent soiling of the lungs with gastric contents. This reflex is lost in the unconscious state.

Pharmacology: anti-emetics, opioids and antacids

CASE 6 (1988–1990)[1]

An obese, anxious woman presented with an ectopic pregnancy of 8 weeks' gestation. Resuscitation, anaesthesia and surgery were uneventful, and her fluid balance was monitored by an internal jugular line. She required a total of 40 mg of papaveretum during the first 6 hours after operation, but was then transferred to patient-controlled analgesia with 4 mg bolus doses of morphine, a 10-minute lockout period and a background infusion of 1 mg/hour. Seven hours later the nurse noted that the patient's breathing was laboured. Three hours after this she was observed to be stuporous and foaming at the mouth. During this 10-hour period she had received a total of 73 mg of morphine. Investigations revealed a PO_2 of 3.6 kPa, a PCO_2 of 5.9 kPa and a WBC of 36,400. A blood culture taken at this time grew Gram-negative bacilli, but these could not be identified. Naloxone and oxygen were administered and the patient was transferred to an ITU, but her chest condition worsened and she died 14 days later from ARDS.

INTERVENTIONS		PROBLEMS
SURGICAL	ANAESTHETIC	
Ectopic pregnancy	General anaesthetic	Uneventful
Postoperative		Papaveretum (large dose) + PCA morphine
		Breathing difficulties
		Stuporous
		Hypoxia
		Gram-negative sepsis
		ARDS

LESSONS

- Sensitivity about pregnancy loss must not prevent proper clinical care.
- Excess opioid usage can obtund consciousness and protective reflexes.
- Close monitoring is necessary when administering analgesia.
- Early detection systems could have prevented deterioration.

CASE 7 (1988–1990)[1]

A young woman required a Caesarean section for an antepartum haemorrhage. She had been given 150 mg of ranitidine orally 6 hours previously. There were no problems with the general anaesthetic, but the patient vomited once in the lateral position when conscious in the recovery area. There was a delay in obtaining crossmatched blood, and the estimated 1.5–2 litres of blood loss was replaced with colloid during the operation, two units of blood being given during the postoperative period. Papaveretum 15 mg was given intramuscularly 1 hour after the end of the anaesthetic, and a further 20 mg were given 80 minutes later. After 2 hours a further 30 mg were given. One hour later the patient was found to be cyanosed and dyspnoeic. Frusemide 40 mg IV was given and the patient was transferred to the ITU, where she died 10 days later from ARDS.

| INTERVENTIONS | | PROBLEMS |
SURGICAL	ANAESTHETIC	
Antepartum haemorrhage Caesarean section	General anaesthetic	Vomited postoperatively
Postoperative		Papaveretum boluses Cyanosis Dyspnoeic

LESSONS

- Silent aspiration may occur in a patient with obtunded reflexes.
- Monitor opioid use, especially in cases where absorption may be impaired (in this case by hypovolaemia).

Knowledge of the neurotransmitters involved in the vomiting reflex has enabled the development of targeted therapy for nausea and vomiting (e.g. dopaminergic, cholinergic, histaminergic and serotonergic antagonists). Treatment of vomiting in pregnancy has been more difficult, due to teratogenicity, as revealed by the adverse effects of thalidomide. Other side-effects are listed in Table 3.2. In addition, the use of dexamethasone in obstetrics remains limited because of lack of evidence regarding fetal safety. Nausea may be experienced during regional anaesthesia, as a result of cerebral hypoperfusion secondary to vasodilation and hypotension, and this is best treated with vasopressors.

Metoclopramide (10 mg 8-hourly, up to 0.5 mg/kg) is the most widely used dopaminergic receptor antagonist.[20–22] At higher doses (up to 5 mg/kg) it also displays serotonin-receptor antagonism. It acts both centrally within the CTZ and peripherally as a prokinetic agent. Gastric motility has complex neural regulation involving stimulation by cholinergic neurons, inhibition by adrenergic neurons, and a complex modulatory influence by dopaminergic and serotonergic neurons. Within the gastrointestinal tract, metoclopramide enhances the motility of smooth muscle from the oesophagus to the proximal small bowel. Thus it accelerates gastric emptying and intestinal transit time, thereby preventing vomiting and reflux. Studies have also reported that metoclopramide significantly increases the mean maximal LOS and barrier pressures (LOS pressure minus intragastric pressure), again decreasing the risk of regurgitation. Its use in obstetrics is long established.[23]

Anticholinergic agents that cross the blood–brain barrier act directly on the vomiting centre to produce their anti-emetic effect. Hyoscine has superseded atropine, but is most effective in the treatment of motion sickness and labyrinthine disease. Antihistamines also act centrally on the vomiting centre, via the vestibular nucleus and nucleus tractus solitarius (e.g. cyclizine). They have prominent anticholinergic side-effects and counteract the emetogenic effects of opioids.

TABLE 3.2 Side-effect profiles of anti-emetic drugs

DRUG CLASS	OTHER RECEPTORS AFFECTED	SIDE-EFFECTS
Dopamine (D_2) antagonists	At high doses, serotonin receptor	Extrapyramidal side-effects, including opisthotonus, oculogyric crisis, dystonia Raised prolactin level Anxiety and depression at high doses
Anticholinergics (ACh)		Blurred vision, dry mouth, urinary retention, confusion
Antihistaminergics (H)	Weak anticholinergics	Anticholinergic effects Drowsiness, insomnia and euphoria Sedative effect enhanced by anaesthetic agents
Serotonin antagonists ($5\text{-}HT_3$)		Relative lack of side-effects – headache, constipation and dizziness Occasional flushing
Proton pump inhibitors (PPI)		Side-effects uncommon – headache, diarrhoea, rashes Dizziness, somnolence, confusion, impotence, gynaecomastia and muscle pains

The serotonergic antagonists, such as ondansetron, were introduced relatively recently. Their effects are mediated by blockade of the $5\text{-}HT_3$ receptor peripherally on vagal afferents and within the vomiting centre. Although many studies have been performed to show the efficacy of ondansetron, there have been few studies of its use in obstetric practice.[24]

An alternative to H_2-receptor antagonists are proton pump inhibitors, such as omeprazole. These are pro-drugs that are activated within the acidic environment of the parietal cells, thus limiting their side-effects to mother and fetus. They non-competitively inhibit gastric acid secretion at the final stage of acid production. Several studies have evaluated the efficacy of proton pump inhibitors for acid aspiration prophylaxis in obstetric anaesthesia.[25] The addition of prokinetic agents appears to be necessary to maximise their effects.

Opioid analgesics are widely used in obstetric practice. Cases 5 and 6 describe excessive administration of these drugs to patients. Pethidine (meperidine) is the opioid of choice during labour for historical reasons, despite its lack of efficacy. In the UK, fentanyl and diamorphine are also frequently used in regional anaesthesia and analgesia. Opioids act centrally via G-protein coupled receptors. Activation results in hyperpolarisation of the membrane potential by potassium ions and suppression of calcium ion flux, thus inhibiting noxious stimuli.

As well as their analgesic effects, opioids exert diverse effects via other systems. Their effects on the gastrointestinal tract are important in parturients. They decrease stomach and intestinal motility. Although the amplitude of non-propulsive rhythmic contractions is enhanced, propulsive contractions are markedly decreased, thus delaying the passage of gastric contents through the duodenum by as much as 12 hours. Studies designed to assess the influence of opioids in labour have shown that women who receive intramuscular opioids, such as pethidine, exhibit delayed gastric emptying and reduced LOS tone. Intrathecal and epidural fentanyl can also delay gastric emptying, and this effect is dose related. Epidural boluses of 50 µg fentanyl and low-dose infusions of local anaesthetic with fentanyl do not appear to delay gastric emptying. Epidural morphine at a dose of 4 mg has been shown to delay gastric emptying.

Histamine (H_2)-receptor antagonists are used in labour to reduce gastric secretions for all high-risk women, and many maternity units give ranitidine in preference to cimetidine.[26–28] This group of drugs competitively inhibits binding of histamine and other H_2 agonists to the H_2 receptor within the stomach. They also prevent acid secretion in response to gastrin and to muscarinic agonists (a lesser agonist). Their net effect is a reduction in the volume of gastric juices and a decrease in hydrogen ion concentration.

Prophylaxis of acid aspiration

CASE 8 (1997–1999)[1]

This patient received five anaesthetics, the first for a Caesarean section during which she suffered a major obstetric haemorrhage. She then required several further operations to control the bleeding. During the fourth operation, abdominal packs were placed to control continuing venous bleeding, and the patient returned to the ICU intubated and ventilated. She was successfully weaned from the ventilator and extubated 24 hours later. Two days later, removal of the abdominal packs was planned. The patient was taken from the ICU to theatre with invasive cardiovascular monitoring in place. There is no record of any gastric secretion prophylaxis prior to this anaesthetic.

After pre-oxygenation, anaesthesia was induced using propofol 120 mg and fentanyl 100 µg. Muscle relaxation was achieved with cisatracurium 14 mg. There was no mention of cricoid pressure. These two facts suggest that a rapid-sequence induction technique was not used on this occasion. Pulmonary aspiration of fluid occurred. The aspirate was tested and gave an acid reaction. Surgery was completed successfully. The patient was extubated and returned to the ICU. Her condition slowly deteriorated and she was re-intubated and required ventilation 24 hours later. Aspiration pneumonitis was subsequently diagnosed on X-ray appearances. The patient continued to deteriorate, and died some 12 days later.

INTERVENTIONS		PROBLEMS
SURGICAL	ANAESTHETIC	
Caesarean section	?General anaesthetic	Major obstetric haemorrhage
Second and third laparotomy	General anaesthetic	To control haemorrhage
Fourth operation	General anaesthetic	Placement of abdominal packs ICU care
Fifth operation	General anaesthetic	No antacid prophylaxis

LESSONS

- Aspiration risk needs to be identified in patients.
- Measures to reduce gastric contents and their acidity and to prevent aspiration should be implemented in patients at high risk of gastric stasis and ileus following multiple abdominal surgery.

CASE 9 (1988–1990)[1]

A young primiparous woman had been admitted to hospital at 35 weeks' gestation with diarrhoea and vomiting thought to be due to gastroenteritis. Shortly after admission she had an eclamptic fit, and the decision was taken to perform an immediate Caesarean section. The patient was given diazepam and chlormethiazole, and was barely conscious on arrival in theatre. She received an uneventful general anaesthetic, but there is no record of the administration of an H_2-blocking drug, or of the stomach being emptied during anaesthesia. The postoperative records are scanty, but it appears that she received 3.5 litres of fluid, of which 2 litres were colloid, during the first 12 hours, although the CVP line was apparently not working. The patient died 10 days later from ARDS.

INTERVENTIONS		PROBLEMS
SURGICAL	ANAESTHETIC	
	Diazepam and chlormethiazole	Eclamptic fit necessitating Caesarean section
Caesarean section	General anaesthetic	Level of consciousness
		Uneventful general anaesthetic
		No record of aspiration prophylaxis
Postoperative		Records scanty
		Inadequate monitoring

LESSONS

- All parturients require adequate antacid prophylaxis.
- Post-ictal patients treated with anticonvulsants have lowered conscious levels, making them vulnerable to regurgitation and aspiration risk.
- Close monitoring of these patients is mandatory peri-operatively.
- Good record keeping is required.
- Patients with eclampsia and pre-eclampsia are vulnerable to fluid overload that may further jeopardise pulmonary reserve. Careful fluid balance is essential.

Since the work of Mendelson and the first CEMD report in 1952 (which had 32 deaths from aspiration in one triennium), a number of strategies have been introduced that have reduced the number of deaths from aspiration. These include the following:
- fasting in labour
- measures to increase gastric pH
- measures to decrease the volume of gastric secretions
- increased use of regional anaesthesia
- use of a rapid-sequence induction (RSI) with a cuffed endotracheal tube (ETT) if a general anaesthetic is required.

Antacids such as magnesium trisilicate were traditionally used in obstetrics. However, between 1994 and 2005 the use of magnesium trisilicate has declined because it produces particulate matter that may worsen the pulmonary 'burn' (chemical pneumonitis) if aspirated.

Other methods of decreasing gastric volume, such as aspiration through a naso-gastric tube or the use of pro-emetic agents, have been advocated by CEMD over the years, although at present such methods are not recommended. Prophylaxis has to cover not only intubation but also extubation and recovery, and is necessary for subsequent surgical interventions.

The implementation of fasting during labour has become controversial. Although pulmonary aspiration is now very rare, it is unlikely that the decrease in its incidence is solely due to restriction of feeding. Midwives argue that labouring women require ingested calories for the increased expenditure of energy during labour, and that restriction of food intake causes discomfort and distress. At present there is little evidence to support either hypothesis. The adverse effect of starvation as shown by an increase in ketones does not appear to be detrimental to either the mother or the fetus. In addition, it has not been shown that starvation affects the duration of labour or the obstetric outcome. However, eating does increase the volume and frequency of vomiting in labour, thus resulting in a significant risk. Several studies have investigated the effect of calorific intake during labour, allowing women to take carbohydrate solutions. The results of these studies have found conflicting effects on the labour outcome. It is hoped that larger randomised controlled studies may be able to find the evidence that is required.

Despite this, there has been an increasing trend towards drinking and eating in labour. In 1988, less than 2% of units in the USA, compared with 33% of units in the UK, were reported to allow solid food intake.[27,28] However, there was no significant increase in cases of mortality in the UK due to aspiration, despite this discrepancy in policies. Subsequent studies have replicated these findings. Of note, one American study of 5,000 women showed that the majority of women preferred to take clear fluids once they were in established labour.[29,30]

Measures to increase gastric pH include the administration of sodium citrate and H_2-receptor antagonists. A number of UK surveys have been conducted each decade to assess current pulmonary aspiration prophylaxis. A 1994 study showed widespread use of 30 ml of 0.3M sodium citrate for Caesarean section, with 90% of elective cases and 99% of emergency cases receiving it.[28] A 2005 study showed a slight decline in citrate use.[27] In contrast, in 1988, 88% of units used ranitidine, whereas in 1994, 57% of units used it prophylactically and a further 16% gave it to 'at-risk' women. In 2005, there was a decline in the number of units using ranitidine before elective Caesarean sections, but there was an increase in administration of the drug to those 'at risk.' The frequency of use of proton pump inhibitors was low, despite evidence for equal efficacy.

Methods of decreasing gastric volume include fasting, enhancing gastric emptying with prokinetic drugs, and decreased use of particulate matter/antacids. Metoclopramide was used as the agent of choice in prophylaxis in approximately 25% of both elective and emergency Caesarean sections in 2005.[27] Antacids tend not to be administered to women at low risk of complications. However, women who have received pethidine (meperidine) during labour have larger gastric volumes, and the use of metoclopramide when pethidine (meperidine) is administered could be beneficial.

The use of regional anaesthesia is not associated with cases of aspiration, unless there are complications such as total spinal blockade or toxicity from local anaesthetics. However, many units continue to use aspiration prophylaxis in patients undergoing Caesarean section, due to the uncertain nature of the surgery and possible conversion to a general anaesthetic.

CHAPTER 4

Regional anaesthesia

MICHAEL KINSELLA, DARYL DOB AND ANITA HOLDCROFT

Maternal deaths from regional anaesthesia have become much more prominent in the last 15 years as a proportion of the total number of anaesthetic-related deaths. This is secondary to a large reduction in mortality from obstetric general anaesthesia, but also because the denominator figures of the number of anaesthetics given has not been taken into account. Between 1982 and 1999 five women died from high spinal (subarachnoid or intrathecal) or total spinal block, and a sixth died as a result of sympathetic nerve blockade associated with inferior vena cava obstruction. In this chapter, the term 'high spinal' has been used to describe a block above the thoracic dermatomes, and the term 'total spinal' when the cranial nerves have been affected. Cranial nerve block does not occur with epidural drug placement, but may occur after either spinal or subdural extra-arachnoid placement. Subdural block is nearly always diagnosed clinically and may have features of both spinal and epidural blocks, leading to confusion and debate about individual cases.[1] Radiographic studies can confirm subdural placement, but may also demonstrate multi-compartment block.[2] Subdural block has not been implicated in any of the CEMD reports from 1982 to 1999.

Systemic toxicity and death resulting from intravenous placement of epidural local anaesthetic have not been described in obstetric practice in the UK. They are inherently less likely now that low-dose solutions are often used. Deaths due to systemic toxicity were recognised in the USA, but have declined in the past decade.[3,4]

The cases

CASE 1 (1982–1984)[5]

One death occurred in association with epidural analgesia. It clearly seems to be a case where the administrative arrangements of the unit were at fault. An epidural block with bupivacaine was instituted by a junior anaesthetist and lasted for around 5 hours. Top-up was delayed until a decision to perform a forceps delivery had been made, and the dose was administered by a midwife, there being no anaesthetist available in this isolated maternity unit. The midwife was called away shortly after administering the dose, and on her return the patient was noted to be blue. Total spinal block was present and cardiac arrest followed. During attempts at resuscitation, the endotracheal tube was misplaced and efficient ventilation was not established before lethal anoxic brain damage had occurred.

The comments by the CEMD were as follows:

The primary failure of care lay in the lack of continued observation following the top-up dose of bupivacaine, because total spinal block should not be lethal. The Standing Advisory Committee on Obstetric Anaesthesia and Analgesia, a joint committee of the Faculty of Anaesthetists of the Royal College of Surgeons of England and the Royal College of Obstetricians and Gynaecologists, recommended that 'in the interests of patient safety, a person proficient in the cardio-pulmonary resuscitation of a pregnant woman should be available within the maternity unit at all times if an epidural is in place.' This policy has been accepted by both bodies.

	INTERVENTIONS		PROBLEMS
SURGICAL	ANAESTHETIC		
Labour	Epidural		
Forceps	Top-up epidural		Midwife top-up
			Midwife called away
	Cardiac arrest and resuscitation		No anaesthetist available
			Endotracheal tube misplaced

LESSONS

■ Midwives should not give individual doses that are associated with a significant risk of high spinal block.

■ Consider restricting midwife top-ups to low-concentration local anaesthetic (e.g. bupivacaine ≤ 0.125%).

■ Ensure that there is continuous observation following top-up.

■ An anaesthetist should be available on site when regional analgesia is in progress.

■ Maintain the cardiopulmonary resuscitation skills of all staff.

CASE 2 (1985–1987)[6]

This woman died more than 6 months after an elective Caesarean section for cephalopelvic disproportion. She had previously had a Caesarean section for cephalopelvic disproportion under general anaesthesia, at which time it had been recorded that tracheal intubation could not be achieved by direct laryngoscopy, and that she had required a blind nasal intubation under inhalational anaesthesia. She was not seen by an anaesthetist until the morning of the planned Caesarean section, and again a consultant anaesthetist was unable to intubate her trachea under direct vision. She was awakened and an epidural anaesthetic was given by an experienced junior anaesthetist who was not directly supervised. A test dose of 2 ml 1% lignocaine was negative, and 8 ml 0.5% bupivacaine was then administered through the epidural catheter. The blood pressure dropped acutely and was maintained with intravenous ephedrine and fluid. There was increasing difficulty in breathing, and spontaneous respiration eventually ceased. Attempts at tracheal intubation were initially unsuccessful, and the tube was then misplaced in the oesophagus. This error was not recognised for some time, but eventually the tube was removed and adequate ventilation was achieved with a mask. Senior anaesthetic assistance had been summoned, and a consultant anaesthetist eventually achieved tracheal intubation. A stillborn infant was delivered by Caesarean section, but the patient suffered severe permanent neurological impairment which resulted in her eventual death.

INTERVENTIONS		PROBLEMS
SURGICAL	ANAESTHETIC	
Previous Caesarean section	General anaesthesia	Difficult intubation
		History not identified until the day of the patient's next Caesarean section
Elective Caesarean section (Grade 4)	General anaesthesia	Unable to intubate
		Patient awoken (consultant involved)
	Epidural planned	Trainee unsupervised
		Inadequate test dose
		No aspiration prior to injection
	Oesophageal intubation	Not immediately recognised
Stillborn baby		Delivery too late

LESSONS

- Aspirate an epidural catheter before injection.
- If surgical anaesthesia is being established, a test dose of the concentrated local anaesthetic should be used (e.g. 3 ml of 0.5% bupivacaine or 2 ml of 2% lidocaine) (not including filter and catheter dead space).
- Allow the test dose time to work.
- A specific management plan should be drawn up during pregnancy for women with a history of difficult intubation, including access to senior help and specialised equipment (*see* Chapter 2).
- Continuing responsibility for the case should include the presence of a consultant once problems have been encountered.
- Always have a plan in case there are unexpected airway difficulties.

Use of a regional technique for Caesarean section in mothers who are known to have a difficult airway is generally advised. Spinal anaesthesia avoids the inherent risks of misplacement of large local anaesthetic doses used during epidural anaesthesia. Concern about a high spinal block can be addressed by the use of an incremental spinal technique, either with a purpose-designed microspinal catheter or intentional spinal placement of an epidural catheter.[7]

Inappropriate test doses are not infrequent in practice.[8] The use of a small dose reduces the risk if placed spinally, but at the expense of a smaller effect that will take longer to manifest and may even be missed. A sensible balance has to be reached. One factor is the site where this is being done. For example, a high or total spinal anaesthetic in a woman who is fully monitored in the operating theatre, correctly positioned, and with resuscitation and delivery facilities immediately available is considerably safer than one that is administered in a labour room. A test dose of 2 ml of 1% lidocaine (20 mg) was given in this case. Although doses as low as 30 mg lidocaine have been shown to provide a demonstrable spinal effect, it is possible that half of the 20 mg dose in this case might have been retained within the epidural filter and catheter unless it was flushed through.

In the UK, it is most common to give concentrated local anaesthetic doses to top up an epidural catheter for operative delivery without using a formal test dose.[8] It is suggested that, in the most urgent cases, waiting 5 to 10 minutes to formally assess a test dose may mean that the epidural block will not be ready sufficiently quickly and general anaesthesia will be required. If the total dose is to be administered as a single bolus, the principles behind the formal test dose can still be applied (i.e. a relatively safe dose of drug should be injected initially, followed by sufficient time for it to have an effect, with close scrutiny of the patient during that period). The suggested doses are 15 mg bupivacaine or 40 mg lidocaine for spinal placement and 25 mg bupivacaine or 100 mg lidocaine for intravenous placement. Spinal or intravenous effects should be apparent within 1 to 2 minutes.

It must be recognised that administration of large doses of local anaesthetic epidurally cannot ever be 100% safe, and facilities for management of high block must always be available (*see* below).

Although the block height was not documented, it is probable that this was a total spinal block. The less likely explanation is that the severe hypotension followed an epidural dose, possibly exacerbated by vena cava compression, resulting in respiratory compromise secondary to cerebral hypoxia. Subsequent difficulties with intubation then compounded the problems.

CASE 3 (1988–1990)[9]

An obese woman was admitted at 30 weeks' gestation for drainage and marsupialisation of a recurrent Bartholin's abscess. The patient asked to be awake during the procedure and agreed to a spinal anaesthetic. She was premedicated with 15 mg of papaveretum, but was very nervous on arrival in the anaesthetic room, her pulse rate being 138–148 beats/min (sinus rhythm), with a normal blood pressure and oxygen saturation. After a pre-load of 400 ml of Hartmann's solution, 1 ml of 0.5% heavy bupivacaine was injected in the sitting position with repeated aspiration of CSF to check that the needle was still *in situ*. After 1 minute the patient noticed some weakness of her legs. She was then placed in the supine position with the head resting on two pillows and the table tilted laterally. Six minutes after injection of the drug the blood pressure was recorded as 102/49 mmHg, with a pulse rate of 159 beats/min, and 2 minutes later the blood pressure had fallen to 75/28 mmHg. The hypotension was treated initially by infusing a further 600 ml of Hartmann's solution and giving two 15 mg doses of ephedrine IV. Shortly after giving the ephedrine, the pulse rate fell to 40–50 beats/min with occasional ectopic beats for about 30 seconds. Oxygen was administered and followed by three doses of 0.6 mg of atropine. Since the hypotension persisted, 1 ml of 1:1,000 adrenaline was given IV. This produced a short period of bigeminy, but 10 minutes after the spinal the blood pressure was 135/86 mmHg and the pulse rate was 104 beats/min. Since the patient had by now received 1000 ml of Hartmann's solution and 600 ml of colloid, the infusion was stopped. Approximately 20 minutes after the spinal injection the patient started to cough up pink, frothy sputum, and had a respiratory rate of 30 breaths/min, a blood pressure of 90/24 mmHg and a pulse rate of 164 beats/min, while the pulse oximeter showed an oxygen saturation of 80%. A total of 60 mg of frusemide (furosemide) was given over the next 10 minutes, and the patient was then given etomidate and suxamethonium to permit tracheal intubation and manual ventilation of the lungs. The abscess was drained and the patient was transferred to the intensive-therapy unit. By the third postoperative day it had become apparent that she had developed severe ARDS, and it was decided that a Caesarean section should be performed to decrease her oxygen requirement. Subsequently, renal failure and disseminated intravascular coagulation developed and continuous inotropic support was required. The patient died 11 days after the spinal anaesthetic. There was no evidence of amniotic fluid embolism or any cardiac abnormality at autopsy.

INTERVENTIONS		PROBLEMS
SURGICAL	ANAESTHETIC	
Incision of abscess	Spinal, sitting position	Tachycardia
	Supine, left tilt	Obesity compounding inferior vena cava obstruction
		Tachyarrhythmia, ephedrine
	Adrenaline 1 ml 1:1000	Profound vasoconstriction + fluid load compromising circulation
		Pink frothy sputum
Abscess drained		
	ITU	
	ARDS	Sepsis (abscess)
Caesarean section		

LESSONS

- Extreme tachycardia is rarely a result of anxiety, but if it is, it should settle with reassurance – if not, consider other causes.
- Consider the possibility of dysrhythmia.
- In the presence of tachycardia, maintain blood pressure by using α-agonists that do not increase the heart rate (e.g. phenylephrine).
- In the presence of cardiovascular collapse after 24 weeks' gestation, position the patient in the full left lateral position if necessary.

In this case, the assessors considered that a tachydysrhythmia might have been mistaken for sinus tachycardia, and that this might have been present without any structural abnormality that would show on autopsy. Intrathecal 0.5% bupivacaine 1 ml in the sitting position is too low a dose to cause a high spinal block. It is possible that the cardiovascular collapse was related to incompletely relieved aortocaval compression despite left lateral tilt. Other speculations consistent with initial sinus tachycardia and subsequent cardiovascular collapse after the regional block include systemic sepsis, pre-eclampsia, pulmonary embolus and phaeochromocytoma.

The CEMD have recommended echocardiography for women when there are symptoms or signs of cardiovascular problems, especially when obesity makes clinical examination difficult.[10,11]

Significant hypotension was treated with intravenous volume replacement and ephedrine. Large doses of ephedrine after spinal anaesthesia in non-obstetric cases have been implicated in the development of coronary artery spasm and myocardial infarction.[12] With the current resurgence of popularity of α-adrenergic agonists in obstetric anaesthetic management,[13] the exclusive use of ephedrine as a vasopressor, as in this case, might be less likely.

In the event of persisting hypotension and bradycardia that are not responsive to fluid administration, first-line management consists of a vasopressor and the lateral position. Adrenaline (epinephrine) is an appropriate second- or third-line vasopressor in doses starting at 5 to 10 μg. However, the dose given in this case (1 ml 1:1000 = 1 mg) is that used for complete cardiac arrest.

With or without any additional medical factors as described above, once pulmonary oedema develops in a pregnant woman this may progress to acute lung injury and ARDS.[14]

CASE 4 (1991–1993)[15]

Thirty-six hours after forceps delivery this patient complained of perineal pain, and epidural analgesia was administered to control this. It appears that the patient was insistent that she did not want an intravenous infusion. She was dehydrated and oliguric, and shortly after epidural insertion she was found to be pale and vasoconstricted. There is no blood pressure record.

The dose of local anaesthetic given is unknown, but it appears that the patient had an extensive block with numbness in her hands. This would have been accompanied by a very extensive sympathetic block, which is poorly tolerated by patients with depleted intravascular volume. The records state that the patient was agitated and restless, but no attempt was made to exclude hypoxia as a cause before giving sedation. Administration of frusemide had no effect on the urine output. No vasopressor medication was given, and no oxygen was administered until an ECG abnormality developed. Hypotension progressed to cardiac arrest. Resuscitation attempts were unsuccessful.

A likely explanation of events is that the extensive epidural block resulted in reduced blood flow to the brain and heart. There may have been additional respiratory depression due to the large dose of epidural opiate. At autopsy the lungs were congested and oedematous and there were two minute emboli in the right lung. There were multiple areas of collapse associated with patchy pulmonary oedema and traces of aspirated vomit in the bronchioles and some alveoli.

	INTERVENTIONS	PROBLEMS
SURGERY	ANAESTHESIA	
Forceps		Dehydrated, oliguric
Perineal pain	Epidural (36 hours after delivery)	No intravenous infusion (Epidural dose not recorded)
		Cardiovascular instability
	Numb hands	Recognition of cervical segmental nerve block
	Restless	Sedation
	Poor urine output	Furosemide given

LESSONS

- Evaluate all body systems prior to giving neuraxial nerve block for pain relief.
- Always establish working intravenous access prior to giving neuraxial nerve block.
- In the event of intravenous access failure (cannula tissues or comes out), and if there is any delay in re-establishing it, use alternative routes for vasopressors – absorption is faster by intramuscular than by subcutaneous route.
- Oxygen, fluids and vasopressors should be given early to hypotensive patients.
- During a regional nerve block, always assume that restlessness is caused by cerebral hypoxia until proved otherwise.

An extensive block in the face of hypovolaemia with no intravenous access or fluid replacement is very likely to produce hypotension. This should be reversed initially with vasoconstrictors, which can be given by routes other than the intravenous one if necessary, followed by fluid replacement that will require intravenous access to be established.

CASE 5 (1994–1996)[16]

A woman of short stature was due to undergo an elective planned Caesarean section, as she was thought to have a big baby and had had a previous Caesarean section for failure to progress in labour. The anaesthetist made several attempts to administer combined spinal and epidural anaesthesia.

This consisted of spinal injection of 2.25 ml heavy bupivacaine, 1.25 µg alfentanil, 150 µg clonidine and 15 ml 0.375% bupivacaine into the epidural space. Shortly afterwards the patient complained of headache, shooting pains down her legs and difficulty with breathing. It was thought that the spinal injection might have been sited a little high, so oxygen was given. The patient's blood pressure fell despite administration of 2.5 litres of fluid and ephedrine, and oxygen saturation deteriorated despite her breathing 100% oxygen. She complained of tightness in her chest and increasing difficulty with breathing, and a decision was taken to intubate and ventilate her. She then developed florid pulmonary oedema. It was decided that she should be transferred to a larger hospital for ventilation. Diuretics and glyceryl trinitrate were given, IV fluids were stopped, central and arterial lines were inserted, and adrenaline was given with midazolam and ketamine for sedation. While waiting for the ambulance the patient deteriorated and had a cardiac arrest. She was given adrenaline and isoprenaline and external cardiac pacing, but could not be resuscitated.

INTERVENTIONS		PROBLEMS
SURGICAL	ANAESTHETIC	
Previous Caesarean section		
Elective Caesarean section	Combined spinal and epidural – multiple attempts	Short stature, big baby
	Spinal	Large doses
	Epidural	Additive effect of epidural drugs
	Fluids 2.5 litres, and ephedrine	Difficulty in breathing, hypotension
?Delivery	Decision to transfer	No transfer

LESSONS

- Assess the patient's stature and the baby's size.
- Combined spinal and epidural anaesthesia allows the flexibility to reduce spinal and epidural doses.
- Epidural solutions, including saline, increase spinal block height.
- Use naloxone to reverse opioid effects if appropriate.
- Consider carefully the rationale for using uncommon adjuvants such as clonidine.

In this case, large doses of anaesthetic were used for the regional blockade in a short woman. The spinal dose was likely to have been sufficient for the operation without the addition of 15 ml of epidural bupivacaine 0.375%. Besides the pharmacological addition of drugs given via these two routes, it is known that expanding the epidural space even with 10 ml of saline increases the height of the spinal block.[17] Furthermore, intrathecal clonidine produces as much hypotension as local anaesthetic, for an equivalent anaesthetic effect.

Current recommendations suggest inserting a spinal needle at L 3/4 or below, in order to reduce the risk of neurological damage,[18] whereas obstetric epidurals are commonly sited one to three interspaces higher. The concern, when problems developed, that the spinal anaesthetic was sited too high may indicate that in this case a needle through needle combined spinal and epidural was inserted at an upper lumbar interspace.

Although the small hole in the dura caused by an obstetric spinal needle will not allow significant transfer of epidural solutions into the spinal space, respiratory arrest or high block may follow accidental dural puncture with the epidural needle.[19] During difficult epidural insertion, it is important to assess the likelihood that unrecognised dural puncture has occurred.

Non-invasive blood pressure measurement is by its nature intermittent, and recordings may be slow or fail completely, with sudden and large changes in blood pressure. Difficulty in breathing was an important initial sign, although it is not specific for respiratory or cardiovascular problems. As in the 1988–90 CEMD report,[9] intravenous fluid and ephedrine failed to reverse hypotension. Effective vasoconstrictors were not given until it was too late to prevent cardiac arrest, and once this has occurred the dose required to re-establish cardiac function may be increased several-fold.[20,21] In this case, maternal position during the collapse is not known, and inferior vena cava compression may have contributed to the events.

CASE 6 (1997–1999)[22]

A woman requested epidural analgesia during her labour. An epidural catheter was sited, but a test dose of 4 ml 0.25% bupivacaine resulted in a high sensory and motor block within 2 to 3 minutes. Clear fluid aspirated from the catheter tested positive for sugar. A diagnosis of subarachnoid catheter placement was made.

It was decided to use the subarachnoid catheter for labour analgesia. All subsequent injections of bupivacaine were given by an anaesthetist, and the quality of the resulting analgesia was described as good. Seven hours later labour had failed to progress, despite oxytocin augmentation, and it was decided to deliver the fetus by Caesarean section. Anaesthesia was not adequate for Caesarean section, so a top-up injection of 2 ml plain bupivacaine 0.5% was given from a 20-ml syringe. The spinal block spread higher than expected. The woman experienced difficulty with breathing and then lost consciousness. She developed a bradycardia of 30 beats/min and the systolic blood pressure decreased to 60 mmHg. The patient was intubated promptly and given fluids, ephedrine, atropine and adrenaline. Cardiac output was restored, but the blood pressure had only increased to 80 mmHg systolic when the baby was born apnoeic and pulseless. The paediatrician had not arrived and the anaesthetist was asked to intubate and resuscitate the baby. By the time the anaesthetist had completed the resuscitation, the obstetrician had discovered an adherent placenta and the mother was losing blood. The obstetrician requested oxytocin (Syntocinon®) to improve uterine tone. The anaesthetist was reluctant to administer this because the systolic blood pressure was only 60 mmHg. After rapid infusion of intravenous colloid solution and further adrenaline, oxytocin 10 IU was given. Cardiac arrest occurred almost immediately. Resuscitation followed accepted practice but was unsuccessful.

| | INTERVENTIONS | PROBLEMS |
SURGICAL	ANAESTHETIC	
Labour	Epidural test dose	High sensory and motor nerve block
	Diagnosed spinal catheterisation	Decision to use catheter
Caesarean section	Inadequate block	?Accuracy of dose
	Top-up	Position not defined
	Difficulty breathing	?Maternal position
	Loss of consciousness	
	Bradycardia (30 beats/min)	
	Hypotension	
Baby born		Paediatrician had not arrived
		Anaesthetist diverted attention to baby
Placenta accreta		Bleeding, hypotension
Oxytocin requested	Fluids, ephedrine and adrenaline before 10 IU oxytocin	Risk of vasodilation with oxytocin

LESSONS

- A spinal catheter after accidental dural puncture will behave differently from a single shot spinal. The drug may enter the CSF much more cephalad because of the interspace used as well as the length of catheter in the space.[23]

- With a background of a pre-existing spinal block, small spinal increments are prudent.
- Intubate promptly if the patient has difficulty breathing and shows cardiovascular collapse.
- Note vasopressor and resuscitation recommendations as before.
- The combination of haemorrhage and a significant anaesthetic problem is unlikely to be manageable safely single-handed. Call for additional anaesthetic support early on.
- Maternal compromise increases the likelihood that neonatal resuscitation will be needed. Call paediatricians early on.
- Note the new recommendations on slow administration of oxytocin.

In this case, lessons from the total spinal death in the previous CEMD (1994–96)[16] appear to have been learned. Difficulty with breathing was again an early sign, followed by bradycardia and hypotension. However, the patient was intubated promptly, and was correctly given ephedrine and adrenaline as vasoconstrictors.

In the event that a severely hypotensive supine woman who is not yet delivered does not respond to these measures, she should be turned to the left lateral position unless delivery can be performed immediately. Relief of inferior vena cava compression in the lateral position or by delivery will usually allow rapid recovery, although once cardiovascular collapse becomes established, recovery may not occur even after restoring venous return in this way.[24] In this case, significant blood loss then ensued before full recovery had occurred. The final precipitant of cardiac arrest in this significantly compromised woman was intravenous administration of oxytocin by bolus.

In obstetric anaesthesia, crises develop rapidly. The request for additional anaesthetic help must be made early on if colleagues are not immediately available on site.

Severe maternal hypotension may well lead to fetal distress and poor physiological state at delivery. It is wise to ensure that paediatric colleagues are advised early on if they might be required for neonatal resuscitation.

Commentary

There were six deaths nationally associated with regional anaesthesia over a 12-year period, five of which were due to high block. There are no denominator data for maternal mortality, but there are reliable figures for the rate of high blocks occurring with regional anaesthesia. In a national survey of anaesthetic techniques used for Caesarean section during 1997, high block was the main cause of serious complications, with regional anaesthesia occurring in 1 in 3,865 cases.[25] In individual series, the incidence of spinal injection or symptomatic high block with epidural blockade is between 1 in 1,374 and 1 in 2,900,[26,27] and the incidence of total spinal or high block requiring tracheal intubation and ventilation is between 1 in 5,498 and 1 in 16,200.[26–28]

In the management of high block, a rapid response to cardiovascular collapse and hypoventilation is crucial. Organisational factors are important for ensuring rapid responses to complications, whether in the delivery room or the operating theatre.

Distribution of spinal solutions

The distribution of injected solutions in the subarachnoid space depends on the dose and volume of the injectate, its baricity, patient position and the physiological changes of pregnancy, as well as position change after the injection. Spinal anaesthesia for Caesarean section requires a mid-thoracic block, and this is usually produced in clinical practice with doses of up to 15 mg of either hyperbaric or plain bupivacaine 0.5%. Doses in this range in volumes of up to 10 ml produce a similar block to concentrated spinal solutions,[29] whereas larger doses – such as may occur with a misplaced epidural top-up – may cause a total spinal block.

Spinal blockade advances cephalad more rapidly in the supine tilted position than in the full lateral position.[30] Head-down tilt will increase the height of the block with hyperbaric solutions unless the upper thorax is also elevated with pillows or by raising the head of the operating table. This position is utilised in the Oxford technique, when the woman's back in the lateral position takes up a 'V' shape.[31] If there are concerns about a high block after a hyperbaric spinal, the benefits of improved venous return with head-down tilt[20] need to be balanced against a possible increase in block height and impaired pulmonary ventilation.

Solutions that are not hyperbaric sometimes have a limited spread within the CSF, but a change in body position may produce a sudden and large increase in block height even 30 minutes after the initial injection.[32] In contrast, a woman who had a large accidental spinal dose of up to 37.5 mg bupivacaine was managed without changing her position, and the block, although profound, did not lead to respiratory compromise.[33]

Relevant cardiovascular physiology

Systemic arterial pressure is the product of cardiac output and systemic vascular resistance. Systemic vascular resistance is generated primarily in the arterioles under the control of the sympathetic nervous system. Basal arteriolar sympathetic tone is highest in the skin and muscle beds, lower in the kidneys, intestine and brain, and least in the heart and lungs.

In the venous system there is active vasomotor control in the splanchnic bed, but very little elsewhere. The central intrathoracic blood volume of approximately 1 litre in a normal adult is contained in the pulmonary vessels, and 80% of this is found in pre- and post-alveolar vessels that are unable to contract. Central blood volume and cardiac filling are dependent on extrathoracic capacitance and resistance vessels.

Acute control of arterial blood pressure occurs through a negative feedback loop mediated primarily by the arterial baroreceptors. These are activated by increases in mean arterial pressure. Afferent stimulation is almost completely absent at a mean arterial pressure of 50 mmHg, and is continuous at 200 mmHg. Arterial baroreceptor activation results in suppression of the sympathetic neurons and activation of the parasympathetic neurons in the brainstem. This results in arteriolar vasodilation and a reduction in heart rate.

Two hormonal systems also aid blood pressure homeostasis. The renin–angiotensin system is stimulated to increase angiotensin levels by low perfusion pressures in the juxtaglomerular apparatus of the kidney. It also responds to increased efferent sympathetic drive via β1-adrenoceptors in the kidneys. Vasopressin is secreted from the posterior pituitary in response to low cerebral perfusion. It is only activated in the presence of significant hypotension.

These arterial pressure control systems primarily regulate the circulation during postural changes, such as moving from the sitting position to standing. However, they will also be activated during bleeding. In healthy subjects, a reduction in blood volume will reduce baroreceptor stimulation. Blood pressure is initially maintained by tachycardia and vasoconstriction. A reduction in arterial pulse pressure indicates that stroke volume is reduced. Arterial pressure is largely maintained until circulating blood volume is reduced by approximately 25–30%.

However, with increasing blood loss there is an increasing likelihood of the appearance of an opposing vasodepressor (vasovagal) response.[20] Although the afferent receptors for this are not fully recognised in humans, the efferent response is the same as baroreceptor stimulation from high arterial pressure. Parasympathetic activation and sympathetic suppression produce 'paradoxical' bradycardia, vasodilation and hypotension. Vasovagal responses are seen in 50% of non-pregnant subjects after blood loss of 1000–1200 ml. Relative or absolute bradycardia in the presence of blood loss must prompt careful assessment of the circulation.

During pregnancy the circulation becomes hyperdynamic, with an increase in cardiac output of 40%, physiological anaemia, and reduced responsiveness to angiotensin. A 20% increase in total blood volume means that blood loss is well tolerated, but vasodilation, warmth of the hands and feet and tissue oedema make it difficult to assess circulating volume deficit, and decompensation may occur abruptly.

The inferior vena cava is usually compressed if a term pregnant woman adopts the supine position, as demonstrated by increases in femoral vein and distal inferior vena cava pressure. Severe compression or even occlusion leads to a reduction in venous return and increased heart rate in about 20–25% of women. Around 5–10% of women develop the supine hypotensive syndrome, often associated with sustained tachycardia but sometimes progressing to bradycardia. Unconsciousness may develop in extreme cases, although a degree of spontaneous recovery can occur. Full resolution is usually rapid on taking up the lateral recumbent position.[30]

Cardiovascular effects of spinal and epidural anaesthesia

Table 4.1 summarises the cardiorespiratory effects of local anaesthetics and opioids administered in the epidural or intrathecal spaces during regional anaesthesia. Adrenaline and local anaesthetics in epidural doses may also produce significant systemic effects even with correct epidural placement.[34] The slow onset of an epidural block gives more time to manage any cardiovascular compromise, such as hypotension or rhythm disturbances. However, in the event of epidural doses of local anaesthetic being delivered spinally, the onset may be rapid, profound and long-lasting.

TABLE 4.1 Cardiorespiratory effects of different segmental levels of regional anaesthetic block and non-segmental sequelae. These are all the consequence of local anaesthetic administration, except for the bottom row. In contrast to solutions administered spinally, epidural administration will not affect the brain or higher cranial nerves, as the epidural space terminates at the foramen magnum

CENTRAL NERVOUS SYSTEM SPREAD	PREDICTED EFFECTS
Brain (cortex, medulla, etc.)	Loss of consciousness, apnoea, cardiovascular depression
Cranial nerves	Facial features of nerve block
Cervical segments (C3–C5)	Diaphragm function lost
Central sympathetic (T1–T4)	'Fixed' slow heart rate
Heart	Horner's syndrome
Stellate ganglion	Loss of vasoconstriction in upper body
	Loss of intercostal muscle function
Abdominal sympathetic (T6–L1)	Loss of cardiac stimulation, reduced circulating catecholamines
Adrenal medulla	
Splanchnic nerves	Loss of vasoconstriction in gut
Peripheral sympathetic (T10–L2)	Loss of vasoconstriction in leg vessels (total systemic vascular resistance maintained)
High block, effects not dependent on segmental level:	
Vasovagal syncope	Bradycardia, vasodilation, hypotension
Effect of severe hypotension, deafferentation	Loss of consciousness, apnoea
Opioid	Sedation, respiratory depression (may be delayed in onset), altered mental status
	Facial features of nerve block

The cardiovascular effects of spinal and epidural anaesthesia are mainly mediated through autonomic efferent block. However, skeletal muscle paralysis also causes failure of the 'muscle pump' in the calves, a mechanism that increases the return of blood to the heart. With increasing doses, spinal anaesthesia will block arteriolar constriction initially in the territory of the sacral roots, then in the legs, trunk and progressing to the arms, beyond which the effects of the higher cervical roots will be negligible. The vasculature of muscle and skin in the limbs accounts for a large amount of systemic vascular resistance. Small volumes of local anaesthetic given epidurally lead to a segmental block that has a defined lower level, but the block required for obstetric surgery extends down to include all of the sacral nerve roots, and is therefore comparable to a spinal in the territories affected. In studies of non-pregnant volunteers, compensatory arteriolar constriction in unblocked areas has been shown to maintain systemic vascular resistance until the block is above T4.[34] Other territories that produce important effects when blocked are the splanchnic nerves T6–L1, causing vasodilation in the gut, blockade of catecholamine secretion from the adrenal medulla and renin from the kidneys, and the cardiac supply at T1–T4, which leads to a reduction in cardiac rate and contractility.

Regional block above T4 is likely to be accompanied by hypotension secondary to reduced systemic vascular resistance.[34] Block to low thoracic levels or above will also impair venoconstriction and the muscle pump. In this situation, the maintenance of passive venous return to the heart by ensuring that the great veins are above the level of the right atrium is critical for cardiac output. Furthermore, a decrease in blood volume may cause circulatory collapse. Bonica and colleagues investigated the effects of removing 10 ml/kg of blood from volunteers who had an epidural blockade to the level of T5 induced with plain lidocaine. In five out of seven subjects, severe cardiovascular depression occurred, necessitating immediate treatment and termination of the study, and two of the subjects had a period of cardiac arrest. Mean arterial pressure decreased to 41% and heart rate decreased to 70% compared with control values.[35]

Spinal and epidural anaesthesia in non-obstetric surgery is associated with an incidence of cardiac arrest of 6 in 10,000 and 1 in 10,000, respectively.[36] Two patterns of susceptibility are present. The first pattern occurs in sick and elderly patients in association with surgical events, and has a poor prognosis. The second pattern occurs in young healthy patients, has a good prognosis, and is attributed to severe vasovagal reactions. The latter occur sometimes, but not exclusively, in the presence of hypovolaemia. Although a distinction between severe vasovagal reactions and cardiac arrest may be arbitrary, it is possible that a delay in active resuscitation of asystole in the presence of regional anaesthesia may decrease the likelihood of success.[37] Resuscitation after cardiac arrest in the presence of regional anaesthesia may be more difficult because of reduced catecholamine release and intrinsic vascular tone.[21] Cardiac arrest in dogs in the presence of an extensive sympathetic block was found to require significantly larger doses of adrenaline than in those without a block, and some could not be resuscitated. Current resuscitation guidelines do not include specific recommendations on vasopressor dose and type for cardiac arrest during regional anaesthesia.

A further factor in some obstetric cases is the presence of inferior vena cava compression by the antepartum uterus. Of the maternal deaths described in this chapter, Case 4 was postpartum, Case 2 had respiratory rather than cardiovascular problems, and Case 3 at 30 weeks' gestation was tilted. In three cases lateral tilt is not mentioned in the vignette. Lateral tilt is often performed inadequately in routine practice.[30] If a 15° tilt is achieved, the effects of inferior vena cava compression are usually negligible in the intact circulation. However, with circulatory collapse, this amount of tilt may not be effective. In recognition of this, the Cardiff resuscitation wedge with a 27° angle was devised for antepartum resuscitation.[38] A purpose-built device such as this will rarely be available in cases of collapse, and tilt or left uterine displacement may have to be applied manually. Once cardiac arrest ensues, relief of the inferior vena cava compression by Caesarean section may be the only way to restore circulation.[38] This is incorporated into international resuscitation guidelines for pregnant women.[39]

Prophylaxis and therapy for cardiovascular effects

A Cochrane Review of techniques aimed at preventing hypotension during spinal anaesthesia for Caesarean section concludes that ephedrine, leg compression and crystalloid prehydration have similar degrees of effectiveness compared with controls (relative risk 0.69–0.78), and that colloid prehydration is approximately twice as effective as crystalloid for the same infused volume.[40] However, recent research on the role of α-adrenergic agonists has changed national practice significantly,[13] although the findings were too recent to be incorporated in this Cochrane Review.

Prehydration

Crystalloid prehydration has been popular for a number of decades, based on favourable results in early trials that have not been replicated. Furthermore, as perception of its limited effectiveness increased, the prehydration volume used increased such that 3–4 litres were given peri-operatively in some regimens. The large capacitance of the venous system allows administration of significant volumes of fluid with little or no increase in arterial pressure. Rapid prehydration just before the spinal anaesthetic increases the CVP to a greater extent than slow prehydration, but with little further benefit in reducing hypotension.[41] Administration of fluid after the spinal anaesthetic has recently been described.[42,43]

Colloid solutions are retained within the circulation much more effectively than crystalloid, and hence have greater effectiveness.[40] They are not often used for prehydration in the UK,[44] possibly because of their greater cost and the small risk of anaphylaxis that is not present with crystalloids.

It is important to recognise from the earlier discussion of cardiovascular interactions between regional anaesthesia and hypovolaemia that blood loss must be aggressively replaced, and that uncorrectable blood volume deficit is a contraindication to high regional anaesthesia.

Leg compression

Leg compression techniques have been studied in a number of randomised controlled trials, but have not been incorporated into routine practice.[40] Their role in resuscitation has not been evaluated.

Vasopressors

Hypotension after regional anaesthesia results from impaired cardiac venous return secondary to altered venous blood distribution, with a lesser contribution from reduced systemic vascular resistance. Blood volume remains unaltered. Vasopressor treatment corrects the change in blood distribution. By increasing systemic vascular resistance, extrathoracic blood volume decreases and up to 300 ml of blood may be infused into the intrathoracic compartment to produce a very rapid increase in cardiac filling.

For many years ephedrine was the only acceptable drug for prophylaxis and treatment of hypotension after obstetric regional anaesthesia. This situation was based on its superiority in preserving uterine blood flow in a sheep model, compared with α-adrenergic agonists during intravenous infusion.[45] However, extensive clinical research has demonstrated that ephedrine is associated with greater neonatal acidosis than are α-adrenergic agonists, probably mediated through direct placental transfer leading to altered fetal metabolism.[46] This effect is dose dependent.[47] Ephedrine as an indirect agonist leads to catecholamine release that stimulates both α- and β-adrenergic receptors, resulting in increased cardiac output in addition to vasoconstriction. However, as a result, tachyphylaxis may occur. Large prophylactic doses may also result in frequent hypertension.[47]

α-Adrenergic agonists act on the peripheral circulation to increase arterial pressure. In contrast to ephedrine, increasing doses of these drugs may reduce neonatal acidosis.[48] Their use is associated with maternal bradycardia, as baroreceptor activation occurs in the absence of direct β-adrenergic stimulation,[46] and with frequent hypertension with high-dose infusions.[43] Some clinicians use α-adrenergic agonists (e.g. phenylephrine) as their first-line vasopressor, and treat bradycardia with anticholinergic drugs,[48] although an alternative approach is to use both ephedrine and an α-adrenergic agonist in variable or fixed combinations.

Bradycardia with α-adrenergic agonists may occur with a normal or rising arterial pressure. However, a combination of bradycardia and hypotension may indicate vasovagal activity. There are no data to suggest whether administration of an α-adrenergic agonist during hypotension with bradycardia will increase heart rate secondary to increased venous return and reduced vasovagal activation, or decrease it further if baroreceptor activity is preserved.

In the event of severe cardiovascular collapse that does not respond rapidly to standard vasopressors, intravenous adrenaline may be required in doses starting at 5 to 10 µg. It has the advantage of achieving powerful vasoconstriction with positive inotropy and chronotropy.

Lateral tilt

Lateral pelvic tilt in the supine pregnant woman is standard practice in obstetric anaesthesia to reduce vena cava compression, but is often inadequately applied. Cardiovascular compensation will counteract residual vena cava compression if the circulation is not severely compromised, but when vasovagal depression occurs, the obstruction to venous return leads to a self-perpetuating cycle. It is essential to increase lateral tilt or use the full lateral position in the presence of persisting severe hypotension while the woman is supine, and prepare for delivery of the fetus in case even this does not produce resolution.[30,39]

Recognition and management of high regional blocks

The potentially catastrophic effects of high regional anaesthesia are fully reversible if well managed.[49] Early recognition of a rising block may prevent morbidity or even mortality. Contributing factors include large epidural doses, multi-compartment block ('catheter migration'), the additive effect of more than one dose into the same or different spaces, and non-hyperbaric solutions given in the sitting position.

Features may include the following:

- weakness and a tingling of the upper arms and shoulders
- difficulty with breathing
- slurred speech or whispering
- sedation
- high dermatomal level of insensitivity to cold and touch.

Although these signs typically occur early, they may develop at a late stage – for example, after operative delivery or Caesarean section when redistribution of blood in Batson's venous plexus of the epidural space occurs. Other features include Horner's syndrome (i.e. a high sympathetic block) and occasionally sixth cranial nerve palsy.

TABLE 4.2 Drill for high regional block in obstetrics[49]

1	Recognise early on. Features may include weakness and/or tingling of the upper arms and shoulders, difficulty breathing, slurred speech and sedation, as well as a demonstrably high level of insensitivity to cold, touch, etc.
	Although typically early and rapidly ascending, symptoms and signs may develop late and insidiously.
2	Call for help.
	Administer oxygen if not already doing so.
	Treat hypotension with uterine displacement, vasoconstrictors (phenylephrine, metaraminol and adrenaline are all suitable in the face of severe maternal hypotension) and intravenous fluids. Maternal blood pressure must be restored to prevent cardiac arrest.
3	Consider the patient's partner. Explain the situation to them and detail a team member to escort them out of the room as soon as possible.
4	Prepare for tracheal intubation if a rapidly ascending block reaches the shoulders or the breathing is affected. Use a rapid-sequence induction with cricoid pressure.
5	Encourage the obstetricians to deliver the baby quickly. This will relieve aortocaval compression.
6	Keep the patient anaesthetised and ventilate the lungs for 1–2 hours. Assess the adequacy of spontaneous ventilation carefully before awakening and tracheal extubation. Remember that peripheral nerve stimulation will not indicate the degree of recession of the block.
7	If intubation is difficult or fails, do not wait for the return of spontaneous ventilation – it may not occur. Go straight to the failed intubation drill.

A high block that requires intubation is a rare event. As a rough estimate, one might be expected each year in a maternity unit that deals with 4,000 deliveries a year. Training in the management of complex but rare problems is most amenable to the 'fire-drill' approach. Table 4.2 is an example of a regional block drill.[49] High regional blocks have been shown to cause 'dissociation', and very small doses of induction agents may be used to induce anaesthesia. Normal doses of induction agents may cause further hypotension in this situation.

In summary, extensive epidural, high spinal or total spinal block is a rare complication that should respond completely to treatment if it is anticipated and dealt with quickly and effectively.

CHAPTER 5

Haemorrhage

BERNARD NORMAN

In the CEMD report for 2000–2002 there were 17 deaths classified as directly due to haemorrhage, 11 deaths due to ectopic pregnancy and one due to genital tract trauma. The number of direct haemorrhage deaths is higher than in recent previous reports due to an increase in the number of cases of postpartum haemorrhage. This increase may be due to the fact that some risk factors are becoming more common. These include increasing maternal age, increasing numbers of women with concurrent medical disease becoming pregnant, and increasing numbers of assisted conception multiple pregnancies. Also, because of the rising Caesarean section rate, there is an increasing risk of placenta praevia and abnormal placental invasion.

Causes of obstetric haemorrhage that feature in the CEMD are listed in Box 5.1. After a section on physiology, these will be discussed below. In order to care for patients with obstetric haemorrhage, the anaesthetist needs to have some insight into obstetric management, so some aspects of this are also covered.

A potentially fatal haemorrhage occurs in 1 in 1,000 obstetric deliveries,[1] and this equates to about 600–700 life-threatening haemorrhages a year in the UK. Only around 1% of these result in a reported death, and it follows that management of obstetric haemorrhage is usually of a high standard. However, the underlying theme in the majority of haemorrhage deaths in the CEMD is substandard care. This is discussed towards the end of the chapter. The chapter concludes with general recommendations for the management of major obstetric haemorrhage.

Physiology of pregnancy and haemorrhage

Pregnancy results in widespread physiological changes to the cardiovascular system.[2] These include the following.

■ Blood volume increases from 70 ml/kg to about 100 ml/kg by term. This increase may be even greater in twin or triplet pregnancies. It is principally caused by an increase in plasma volume, but there is also a variable rise in the total volume of circulating red blood cells.

■ Haemoglobin concentration decreases, often to about 12 g/dl by term. This is

---

BOX 5.1 Causes of obstetric haemorrhage

Early pregnancy
- Miscarriage and termination of pregnancy
- Ectopic pregnancy

Antepartum haemorrhage
- Placental abruption
- Placenta praevia
- Spontaneous uterine rupture

Postpartum haemorrhage
- Abnormal placental invasion
- Uterine atony
- Surgical misadventure
- Genital tract trauma
- Extrauterine pregnancy
- Retained placenta or placental fragments

Other
- Refusal of blood and blood products
- Coagulopathy

---

because the increase in plasma volume is greater than the rise in the number of red blood cells.

- Cardiac output increases by about 50% by term. This is mediated by a rise in stroke volume of around 25% and an increase in heart rate of around 20%.
- Respiratory tidal volume increases by 45% during pregnancy, causing a similar increase in minute volume (the respiratory rate is largely unchanged). This causes a reduction in PCO_2. However, this fall is matched by an increase in renal bicarbonate excretion, so that blood pH shows little change.
- The rise in tidal volume and cardiac output ensures that there is increased oxygen delivery to the tissues despite the reduced haemoglobin concentration. Oxygen consumption increases by 40–60% in pregnant women.
- Systolic and diastolic blood pressures decrease in early to mid gestation, but return to normal at term.
- Systemic vascular resistance (SVR) is proportional to blood pressure divided by cardiac output. Therefore SVR decreases as the cardiac output increases in pregnancy. It is 20% below non-pregnant levels at term.
- Uterine blood flow increases from about 100 ml/min before conception to 700–900 ml/min at term. This flow is mainly from the internal iliac arteries via the uterine and, to a lesser extent, vaginal arteries. However, there is also an extensive collateral circulation to the uterus. The uterine arteries anastomose with the ovarian arteries, which take their supply from the abdominal aorta,

while other branches of the internal iliac arteries anastomose with branches of the external iliac and inferior mesenteric arteries.

■ Pregnancy is a hypercoagulable state – there is an increase in the concentration of many clotting factors as well as an increase in platelet activation. The hyper-coagulability probably helps to reduce haemorrhage. This may explain why obstetric haemorrhage can become particularly severe when this situation is reversed and a coagulopathy develops.

The increase in blood volume and cardiac output in pregnancy may result in the signs of haemorrhage presenting relatively late. Tachycardia may be the only sign of haemorrhage until 30–40% of the blood volume has been lost. In addition, some patients may be bradycardic rather than tachycardic. This may be due to increased vagal tone.[3] Patients on β-adrenergic blockers for pregnancy-induced hypertension will also fail to mount a normal tachycardic response. Accuracy of blood pressure measurement may present further problems in these cases. For example, staff may focus on the diastolic pressure, which is a derived value when measured by automated devices.

In addition to the variable blood pressure and heart rate changes discussed above, occult haemorrhage may present with anxiety, pallor, sweating, tachypnoea, decreased urine output, a decrease in the volume of the pulse oximetry trace or difficulty in obtaining a pulse oximetry reading. Published texts on haemorrhage often contain tables showing how clinical signs change with increasing blood loss.[4,5] However, they are not representative of the presentation of every case, especially if one focuses purely on one or two parameters. The difficulty of diagnosing obstetric haemorrhage on the basis of clinical signs is illustrated in the following vignette.

CASE 1 (1994–1996)[6]

A parous woman in the third trimester was admitted to an Accident and Emergency department at night because she was feeling unwell. She was noted to be pale and clammy, but she was not in pain and her pulse and blood pressure were normal. She was placed in a cubicle and was thought to be asleep. When the doctor saw her, just 2 hours after admission, she was found to be dead. Her haemoglobin was 3.0 g%. At emergency Caesarean section the uterus contained 2 litres of blood.

Clearly this patient was not just a victim of her physiology. The CEMD were critical of her care. They advised that any pregnant woman admitted to an Accident and Emergency department should be discussed with the duty obstetrician. However, this case does demonstrate that hypovolaemia can be relatively occult in a pregnant woman.

Miscarriage and termination of pregnancy

Both miscarriage (with retained products of conception) and termination of pregnancy can result in haemorrhage. However, only one such death was reported between 1994 and 2002, and this is described in the following vignette.

CASE 2 (1997–1999)[7]

A woman suffered an early fetal loss and was anaesthetised for evacuation of retained products of conception by a junior trainee anaesthetist. Following the surgery, the woman continued to lose blood per vaginum. On return to theatre, she was again anaesthetised by a junior anaesthetist. Consultant input into her care did not begin for another hour. She eventually underwent hysterectomy. During the operation she suffered further major haemorrhage, but blood replacement was limited to 5 units of blood. Maintenance of her blood pressure required methoxamine and noradrenaline/norepinephrine throughout the operation. Transfer to the ICU was intended, but while being moved to her bed the patient arrested. Although she was resuscitated, she died shortly afterwards in the ICU.

The CEMD commented that in this case there had been over-reliance on vasoconstrictors rather than blood transfusion to maintain blood pressure. In addition, the delay in involvement of a consultant anaesthetist was substandard.

Ectopic pregnancy

There were 11 deaths due to ectopic pregnancy reported in the CEMD report for 2000–2002, of which eight sought medical care. This is similar to the figures in previous reports. In 4 of the 11 cases the ectopic pregnancy was in the portion of the Fallopian tube within the wall of the uterus. This type of ectopic pregnancy is called a cornual or interstitial pregnancy. Interstitial pregnancies account for a small proportion of ectopic pregnancies but have a high mortality rate.[8]

Anaesthetic care was not always good in the cases of ectopic pregnancy reported, and sometimes attempts to restore a normal blood volume inappropriately delayed transfer to the operating theatre for definitive surgical treatment. However, the principal problem was delay in diagnosis. In all of the cases reported in 2000–2002 there was a failure to make the diagnosis prior to rupture. Women with ectopic pregnancies may have symptoms that suggest gastrointestinal or urinary tract problems. Therefore all women of reproductive age attending with abdominal symptoms should have a pregnancy test.

Placental abruption

There have been three or four deaths from placental abruption in each of the CEMD triennial reports from 1991 to 2002.

CASE 3 (1997–1999)[9]

A woman with a known history of domestic violence and drug abuse lived in poor social circumstances. She had been diagnosed late in the second trimester as having pulmonary hypertension secondary to possible subacute bacterial endocarditis. Appropriate plans were made for her delivery, but she was admitted in hypovolaemic shock several weeks later, with clear evidence of abruption of the placenta and of right heart failure. There were also signs of bruises on her abdomen and arms. As there was fetal distress, a rapid Caesarean section was performed for the benefit of both the baby and the mother. The baby survived, but the mother could not be resuscitated from cardiogenic shock, despite the presence of three consultant anaesthetists, one of whom had previously assessed the patient.

Risk factors for placental abruption include the following:
- first pregnancy
- abruption in previous pregnancy
- hypertension
- placental dysfunction (including pre-eclampsia)
- prolonged rupture of membranes
- abdominal trauma
- cocaine abuse.

It is likely that the patient in the above vignette had more than one of these risk factors. It is not known whether she also took cocaine. Cocaine causes hypertension and uterine vasoconstriction, which can trigger placental abruption.[10]

Although not a feature in the above vignette, a substantial proportion of placental abruption deaths are associated with an underestimation of blood loss. This is because the haemorrhage may be retroplacental and therefore concealed. In addition, abruption is often complicated by disseminated intravascular coagulation (DIC). This is discussed later in the chapter (*see* page 101).

Placenta praevia and abnormal placental invasion

Box 5.2 gives details of placenta praevia and the different types of abnormal placental invasion (placenta accreta, increta and percreta).

There have been three or four deaths from placenta praevia (with or without

BOX 5.2 Placenta praevia and abnormal placental invasion[4]

Placenta praevia

The placenta is close to or lies over the cervical os. Diagnosis is by ultrasound scanning. Placenta praevia can cause bleeding (sometimes severe) from the placental bed both before and at the time of delivery. There are four grades, and the higher grades require Caesarean section.

- Grade 1. The placenta is within the lower uterine section but does not reach the internal os.
- Grade 2. The placenta reaches the os.
- Grade 3. The edge of the placenta covers the os.
- Grade 4. The centre of the placenta covers the os.

Abnormal placental invasion

There are three types.

- Placenta accreta (78% of cases). The placenta is abnormally adherent to the uterine muscle. It is difficult to diagnose using ultrasound scanning. The placenta fails to separate easily from the uterus after delivery, and there is often severe bleeding.
- Placenta increta (17% of cases). The placenta has invaded the uterine muscle, causing similar difficulties to placenta accreta. It can often be diagnosed using ultrasound scanning.
- Placenta percreta (5% of cases). The placenta has penetrated through the uterine muscle and into structures beyond the uterus, such as the bladder wall. Like placenta increta, it can often be diagnosed using ultrasound scanning. It causes very severe bleeding after delivery.

Abnormal placental invasion is usually associated with placenta praevia, particularly after previous Caesarean sections when the placenta praevia lies in an anterior position over the scar. If there is placenta praevia, the risk of placenta accreta is 5%, 10% or 60%, depending on whether the mother has had no, one or more previous Caesarean sections, respectively.

abnormal placental invasion) in each of the CEMD triennial reports from 1991 to 2002. Caesarean section increases the likelihood of these conditions occurring in subsequent pregnancies. While the Caesarean section rate is high, these conditions will continue to be a significant cause of mortality.

Placenta praevia is usually classified as a cause of antepartum haemorrhage. However, in the majority of cases reported, the life-threatening haemorrhage occurred following the Caesarean delivery that the placenta praevia required. Usually there was an abnormally adherent placenta and the bleeding was severe, as illustrated by the following vignette.

CASE 4 (1997–1999)[9]

A multiparous woman who had had a number of previous Caesarean sections (the first for strong fetal indications, and the following ones elective) was diagnosed as having placenta praevia on ultrasound scan at about 20 weeks' gestation. She had recurrent episodes of bleeding from then onwards. The risk of placenta accreta and major haemorrhage was repeatedly discussed with the woman and among all of the relevant staff, and detailed multi-disciplinary plans were made for a planned Caesarean section at 36 weeks, and for an emergency section should bleeding or labour occur before this. Heavy bleeding, in the early hours of the morning, did occur just before the planned section, and the prepared plan was immediately put into action. Surgery, including Caesarean section, a hysterectomy and cross clamping of the aorta was performed by three consultant obstetricians and a consultant vascular surgeon. The consultant anaesthetist was fully supported by staff from the ICU, and extra experienced midwifery and theatre staff were on duty. A total of 60 units of blood were given in the first 2 hours, and 200 units were given altogether. After a few hours the situation appeared to be temporarily stable and the patient was transferred to the ICU. Unfortunately, further bleeding occurred and she eventually died a few weeks later without recovering consciousness.

It is thought that this patient had placenta percreta. The CEMD describes her care as exemplary. Unfortunately, this is unusual. Contributing factors to other placenta praevia deaths reported by the CEMD include inexperienced anaesthetists and surgeons, failure to secure adequate venous access prior to delivery, delivery in isolated sites without an on-site blood bank, and failure to use CVP monitoring.

Women with placenta praevia after a previous Caesarean section are known to be particularly at risk of haemorrhage. Ultrasound scanning allows the diagnosis of placenta praevia to be made well in advance of delivery, so staff should be aware of the risk of severe bleeding. An advance plan of management and adequate preparation for a major haemorrhage at the time of delivery are essential. Box 5.3 lists the recommendations for the management of women known to be at risk of obstetric haemorrhage, and is modified from the CEMD report for 1997–99. The CEMD 2000–2002 report recommends that the insertion of bilateral iliac artery balloon catheters immediately prior to Caesarean section should be considered in elective cases at high risk of placenta accreta.

Spontaneous uterine rupture and other genital tract trauma

There has been a decrease in the number of deaths from spontaneous uterine rupture in recent years, despite the increase in the number of mothers who have had previous

Caesarean section. There were four cases in 1994–96, one in 1997–99, and none in 2000–2002.

CASE 5 (1991–1993)[11]

A grand multiparous woman was booked for confinement in a general practitioner maternity unit. Her past obstetric history had been uneventful. Labour was induced with prostaglandin pessaries, as the pregnancy was post-term. She had a normal vaginal delivery. Approximately 1 hour later she complained of breathing difficulties, collapsed and failed to respond to resuscitative measures. At autopsy a large quantity of blood was present in the abdominal cavity, and there was a rupture on the left side of the lower uterine segment.

BOX 5.3 Recommendations for the management of women known to be at risk of obstetric haemorrhage[9]

In cases where a delivery is known to be associated with a higher risk of major bleeding – for example, placenta praevia, especially with previous Caesarean section, myomectomy scars, uterine fibroids, placental abruption or previous third-stage complications – the following steps are essential.

- Possible prepartum anaemia should be checked and corrected in the antenatal period if possible.
- All elective or emergency surgery should be performed by a consultant.
- Any anaesthetic should be given by a consultant.
- Adequate intravenous access (two or more cannulae, minimum size 16 gauge) should be in place before surgery starts.
- At least 4 units of blood should be crossmatched and immediately available.
- A central venous pressure line should be in place, either pre-operatively or whenever it is apparent that bleeding is excessive.
- If bleeding is excessive, the obstetrician should consider either embolisation of uterine arteries by an interventional radiologist or further surgical procedures, such as internal iliac ligation, hysterectomy or B-Lynch suture. (These techniques are discussed further on pages 97 and 109.) Any obstetrician who does not feel competent to perform any of the above should immediately call a colleague to assist or, if necessary, a vascular surgeon.
- The advice of a consultant haematologist should be sought to assist in the management of coagulopathy (e.g. due to disseminated intravascular coagulation or massive transfusion). The most appropriate blood product replacement is dependent on the results of coagulation tests and full blood count, and may involve cryoprecipitate, fresh frozen plasma and platelets (*see* page 106).

This patient had at least two risk factors for uterine rupture. Risk factors include the following:

- previous Caesarean section or other uterine surgery (such as myomectomy)
- induction of labour (especially if multiple doses of prostaglandin are used)
- augmentation of labour with oxytocin
- cephalopelvic disproportion
- multiple previous pregnancies.

Fetal stress, as indicated by abnormalities of the fetal heart rate, is common when uterine rupture occurs. Likewise, although uterine rupture sometimes occurs before labour and can sometimes be painless, it usually occurs during labour and is associated with severe pain. An anaesthetist who sees a labouring woman in pain despite a functioning epidural should consider a uterine rupture, especially if the fetal heart trace is abnormal or the patient has any of the above risk factors.

Genital tract trauma other than that due to spontaneous uterine rupture has accounted for three deaths between 1994 and 2002. Two of them followed a forceps delivery. Sometimes genital tract trauma bleeding can be concealed – for example, if there is a retroperitoneal haematoma. The CEMD 2000–2002 report advises that for all types of genital tract trauma, urgent and skilled intervention is needed, and that a consultant obstetrician performing a hysterectomy for genital tract trauma should have support available from another consultant.

Uterine atony

Uterine atony (failure of the uterus to contract after delivery) is associated with multiple gestation, macrosomia, polyhydramnios and high parity. It is the commonest cause of postpartum haemorrhage and the most likely indication for peripartum blood transfusion.[12] However, in isolation it is rarely a cause of fatal obstetric haemorrhage, although it often complicates other causes of haemorrhage. Between 1994 and 2002 there has been only one death from uterine atony, and this may have been caused by sepsis, as described in the following vignette.

CASE 6 (1994–1996)[6]

An older primigravid woman with a fear of hospitals went into labour at home at 39 weeks' gestation after normal antenatal care. She was transferred to hospital because of a delay in the second stage, and vacuum extraction was performed because of fetal distress. One hour after delivery the patient's temperature was 38.2°C. At 2 hours she felt unwell and at 3 hours she collapsed with a massive atonic postpartum haemorrhage. The platelet count was 36,000. The patient was anaesthetised and underwent laparotomy 2 hours later. There was 'offensive' free fluid in the peritoneal cavity. She died several hours after delivery.

BOX 5.4 Management of uterine atony

Pharmacological options

- Ergometrine (500 µg slowly IV, or 500 µg IM in combination with oxytocin 5 units)
- Oxytocin (5 units slowly IV, then 40 units over 4 hours)
- Carboprost (250 µg IM, may be repeated up to 8 times at a minimum of 15-minute intervals; alternatively, can be given intramyometrially at the same dose)
- Misoprostol (1 mg rectally)

Mechanical manoeuvres

- Uterine massage to stimulate contraction
- Bimanual compression of uterus
- Balloon compression device inserted into uterus (Cook's catheter)
- Aortic compression with fist above umbilicus directed backward against spine

Surgical options

- Examine in theatre under anaesthesia to exclude or treat retained placental fragments or genital tract trauma
- Packing of the uterine cavity
- Hysterectomy
- B-Lynch suture
- Uterine artery or internal iliac artery ligation
- Cross clamping of the aorta (by a vascular surgeon) to control bleeding prior to definitive surgical management

The fact that uterine atony is rarely fatal may reflect generally good practice in its treatment. Box 5.4 lists the options for its management (including drug doses), and further details of these treatments are discussed below.

Pharmacological options

Ergometrine, which is an ergot alkaloid derived from a fungus, is a uterine muscle stimulant. Its side-effects include nausea, vomiting and vasoconstriction. The vasoconstriction results in an increase in blood pressure that lasts for several hours and can be hazardous in pre-eclampsia and heart disease. Ergometrine is often given in combination with oxytocin at the end of the second stage of labour as prophylaxis against uterine atony.

Oxytocin is a hormone secreted by the posterior pituitary. It binds to receptors on smooth muscle in the uterus and milk ducts, stimulating contraction. The synthetic preparation now used is vasopressin-free, unlike the older pituitary extract preparation. Compared with ergometrine, oxytocin causes less nausea and vomiting and also produces hypotension rather than hypertension. The hypotension is due to a substantial decrease in systemic vascular resistance caused by oxytocin. There is a compensatory tachycardia which is particularly marked if a large bolus is given. Paradoxically, oxytocin increases pulmonary artery pressure. Because of its cardiovascular effects, oxytocin should only be given to patients with cardiac disease very slowly and at a low dose, if at all.

Carboprost is a prostaglandin analogue (prostaglandin $F_{2\alpha}$) which increases myometrial intracellular calcium and so causes uterine contraction. It is indicated in patients with uterine atony that is not responsive to ergometrine and oxytocin. Side-effects include vomiting, diarrhoea, fever and bronchospasm.

Misoprostol is also a prostaglandin analogue (prostaglandin E_1) that is used to stimulate uterine contraction when other measures have failed. Like carboprost, its side-effects include vomiting and diarrhoea. Despite being an effective treatment for uterine atony, it is not licensed for this indication – its licensed use is to prevent or treat peptic ulcers.

Mechanical manoeuvres

These may be of value in reducing haemorrhage. Uterine massage often stimulates contraction, and may be the only treatment required for mild uterine atony. If this fails, pressure on the uterine placental bed may reduce haemorrhage and be a useful holding measure until definitive treatment can be given. This can be achieved by bimanual compression of the uterus, or using a balloon compression device inserted into the uterus, such as a Cook's catheter. Reducing the blood flow to the uterus by aortic compression is also an option. This is achieved using a fist above the umbilicus directed backwards against the spine.

Surgical options

If the patient is not already undergoing surgery, there should be a low threshold to examine the patient in theatre under anaesthesia to exclude or treat retained placental fragments or genital tract trauma. Care should be taken to avoid using unnecessarily high concentrations of volatile anaesthetic agents, as these relax uterine muscle and make uterine atony worse. Surgical manoeuvres to treat atony include packing the uterine cavity to compress the bleeding placental bed, hysterectomy or B-Lynch suture. The B-Lynch suture is a continuous 'brace' suture through the full thickness of the intact uterus. This compresses the uterus and so reduces bleeding. Its use was first reported in 1997, and it is now gaining acceptance as an alternative to hysterectomy in the surgical management of postpartum haemorrhage.[13] Another option is ligation of the uterine or internal iliac arteries. However, because of the collateral blood flow to the uterus, as described early in the chapter, this often has only a marginal effect on blood loss. Finally, in extremis, a vascular surgeon can be asked to cross clamp the aorta to control bleeding prior to definitive surgical management.

Surgical misadventure

Ten of the postpartum haemorrhage cases reported by the CEMD between 1991 and 2002 have been associated with surgical misadventure, usually during Caesarean section.

CASE 7 (1994–1996)[6]

A woman who had undergone two previous Caesarean sections was booked for an elective Caesarean section at 38 weeks' gestation. She was admitted in spontaneous labour 2 days before that date, and Caesarean section was performed by a registrar. 'Some bleeding' was noted from the angle of the uterine incision. Twenty-one hours after the operation the patient collapsed on the postnatal ward. Laparotomy revealed a retroperitoneal haematoma. Hysterectomy was performed by two consultants and the patient was transferred to an ICU in another hospital. At a further laparotomy a 2-mm tear in the iliac vein and a 1-cm laceration in the liver were repaired. The patient was returned to the ICU but died the next day.

In this case, care was considered to be substandard, as an unsupervised registrar was operating on a patient who had had two previous Caesarean sections. Bleeding from surgical misadventure does not necessarily equate to substandard care. However, of the 10 cases reported between 1991 and 2002, none were noted as having their initial surgery performed by a consultant.

Extrauterine pregnancy

There has been only one death due to extrauterine pregnancy between 1991 and 2002, as described in the following vignette.

CASE 8 (1991–1993)[14]

This patient's past history included appendicitis, a pelvic abscess and several laparotomies for adhesions. She had experienced repeated episodes of abdominal pain (and indeed underwent laparotomy for suspected ectopic pregnancy), but subsequent ultrasound scans suggested an intrauterine pregnancy. An elective Caesarean section was planned for an unstable lie, but at operation an extrauterine pregnancy was found. There was heavy bleeding when the placenta was removed. Blood was transfused, but cardiac arrest occurred in the ICU.

In advanced extrauterine pregnancy the placenta should be left in place after the baby has been delivered at laparotomy, as attempts to remove the placenta can, as in this case, cause uncontrollable bleeding.

Retained placenta or placental fragments

Both retained placenta and placental fragments (products of conception) can cause life-threatening haemorrhage. Between 1991 and 2002 there was one reported death due to each. The patient who died because of bleeding due to a retained placenta received substandard care.[9] Although she was a high-risk patient, she was induced at a weekend in a hospital without an on-site blood bank, and when haemorrhage occurred there was a delay in calling obstetric staff. In contrast, the patient who died because of bleeding due to retained placental fragments was well cared for (*see* Case 9).

Refusal of blood and blood products

CASE 9 (1991–1993)[14]

Eight days after a normal vaginal delivery a woman underwent uterine curettage for retained products of conception. Three days later she was readmitted with secondary postpartum haemorrhage, and a further uterine evacuation was performed. She continued to bleed during the operation. The consultant anaesthetist attended and the consultant obstetrician performed a hysterectomy. The patient died 4 hours after the hysterectomy.

This patient died because she refused a blood transfusion despite clear and repeated warnings about the risk of death.

Between 1982 and 2002 there were six cases of death in women who refused blood transfusion because of personal or religious beliefs. The CEMD 2000–2002 report contains guidelines for the management and treatment of obstetric haemorrhage in such women. A synopsis is given in Box 5.5. The effect on the staff caring for such women can be devastating, as these deaths should be preventable.

Coagulopathy

Severe obstetric haemorrhage is often further complicated or even caused by coagulopathy. If coagulopathy is the principal cause of haemorrhage, the haemorrhage often follows Caesarean section necessitated by either pre-eclampsia or sepsis. An example of the latter is given in the following vignette.

CASE 10 (1997–1999)[9]

A woman with septicaemic shock and an intrauterine death developed DIC secondary to sepsis from group-A haemolytic streptococcus. The seriousness of her condition was not recognised until several hours after admission, when she was *in extremis*. Resuscitation was then undertaken, but the treatment of DIC was delayed because the laboratory was not on site and platelets had to be sent from 60 miles away. A few hours after admission, because delivery was not imminent, a Caesarean section was performed in case the sepsis was intrauterine, although this proved not to be the case. After the operation, the DIC and vaginal bleeding persisted and the patient was transferred to an ICU, where she received a total of 56 units of blood, 36 units of fresh frozen plasma, 13 units of platelets and 14 units of cryoprecipitate. Her condition did not improve and her uterine arteries were embolised the next day, but this did not provide any long-term benefit. Antibiotic treatment was inhibited by a history of penicillin allergy.

BOX 5.5 Management and treatment of obstetric haemorrhage in women who decline blood transfusion[15]

Antenatal care
- At booking, establish the patient's wishes with regard to blood transfusion and cell salvage (collecting blood from the operative field and re-infusing the red blood cells).
- If necessary, refer the patient for care in a unit where interventional radiology and cell salvage are available.

Labour
- As vaginal delivery is usually associated with less blood loss than Caesarean section, the latter should be performed only for a clear indication and by a consultant obstetrician.
- Oxytocics should be used for the third stage of labour.

Haemorrhage
- If bleeding does occur, there should be a low threshold for using physical and pharmacological methods to stem it.
- Physical methods include uterine artery embolisation (if the patient is stable enough for transfer to the radiology department), B-Lynch suture, internal iliac ligation and hysterectomy.
- Pharmacological methods include intravenous vitamin K and antifibrinolytics such as tranexamic acid.
- Cell salvage should be used if possible.
- If the situation is critical, the woman should if possible be asked again to accept blood transfusion. This should not be done in the presence of relatives or her partner, who may decrease the likelihood of her making a choice of her own free will.

This case illustrates the importance of prompt diagnosis of coagulopathy, and the value of having a blood laboratory on site in high-risk cases.

Coagulopathy associated with obstetric haemorrhage is usually of one or more of the following types.

Dilutional coagulopathy

This occurs when one to one and a half times the blood volume has been transfused, and is due to loss of clotting factors and platelets.

Disseminated intravascular coagulation (DIC)

This pathological activation of coagulation is often triggered by obstetric causes and frequently complicates obstetric haemorrhage. Details are given in Box 5.6. Unfortunately, DIC has a poor prognosis and is difficult to manage.[16]

BOX 5.6 Disseminated intravascular coagulation (DIC)[16–18]

Obstetric causes of DIC
- Amniotic fluid embolism
- Pre-eclampsia and HELLP
- Placental abruption
- Obstetric haemorrhage
- Intrauterine death
- Retained products of conception
- Sepsis

Pathology
Pathological activation of coagulation results in:
- fibrin clot formation
- consumption of platelets and clotting factors, causing coagulopathy
- secondary fibrinolysis, also causing coagulopathy
- fibrin deposition in small vessels, causing organ failure.

Diagnosis
Clotting screen has widespread abnormalities, often with fibrin degradation products such as D-dimers.

Treatment
- Remove the underlying cause.
- Use supportive measures to maintain tissue perfusion and oxygenation.
- Keep the patient and transfused fluids warm, as hypothermia increases coagulopathy.
- A consultant haematologist should guide haematological management. This will include administration of fresh frozen plasma, platelets and possibly cryoprecipitate or protein C.

Haemolysis, elevated liver enzymes, low platelets (HELLP)

This syndrome may cause a coagulopathy due to DIC and thrombocytopenia. It is discussed in Chapter 6.

Coagulopathy secondary to anticoagulation

The CEMD 1997–99 report describes the death of a woman who was anticoagulated because of a familial tendency to venous thrombosis, and who suffered haemorrhage before and after surgical repair of a uterine rupture.[19] The CEMD recommend careful haemostasis in fully anticoagulated patients who are having surgery, and conversion to heparin to allow reversal with protamine sulphate if required.

The treatment of all types of coagulopathy is the same as that outlined for DIC in Box 5.6. Specific guidance on the administration of blood components is given later in the chapter, in Box 5.9. Involvement of a consultant haematologist in the management of coagulopathy is particularly important, and is emphasised in the CEMD 2000–2002 report.

Substandard care

Death from obstetric haemorrhage is often associated with substandard care. There were 17 direct haemorrhage deaths reported between 2000 and 2002. In two of these cases there was no contact with medical services. Of the 15 deaths where medical care had been sought, four-fifths (12 cases) received substandard care, and one-third (5 cases) received substandard anaesthetic care. A similar incidence of substandard care has been reported in previous years. The following case is typical.

CASE 11 (1997–1999)[7]

This patient had a medical history that included bicornuate uterus, uterine surgery to correct it, previous Caesarean section and a recognised placenta praevia in the current pregnancy. She spent the last weeks of her pregnancy as an inpatient. She had a pre-operative haemoglobin level of 9.1 g/dl and was clearly a very high-risk patient. The obstetric service had more than a month in which to make the necessary consultations and arrangements to ensure consultant anaesthetic involvement for the planned elective Caesarean section. However, contact with the anaesthesia service was delayed until the day before the planned operation, because the surgeon did not anticipate problems. Two inexperienced trainees provided anaesthesia because there was no consultant available on the day of the operation. A general anaesthetic was given using a standard technique. The case was apparently started with only one peripheral intravenous cannula sited. Surgery was uneventful until a major haemorrhage occurred. According to the anaesthetists, the woman suffered blood loss of 6.5 litres. Despite the major blood loss and limited venous access, initial resuscitation was ultimately successful. However, the patient was hypotensive for 45 minutes, and the lack of CVP monitoring must have made it difficult to judge the adequacy of fluid replacement. The patient was transferred from theatre to the high-dependency unit, where she suffered further blood loss, necessitating laparotomy. She died shortly after induction of anaesthesia for this surgery.

It is interesting to compare this case with Case 4, given earlier in the chapter in the section on placenta praevia and abnormal placental invasion. In Case 4, care was good. In Case 11, care was substandard in several respects. There was poor inter-specialty communication, no consultant anaesthetist, inadequate venous access, no CVP monitoring and probably inadequate blood volume replacement.

Box 5.7 lists the recurring aspects of substandard care that are reported in the CEMD reports. Many of them will be familiar to obstetric anaesthetists, and examples are to be found in many of the preceding vignettes. Most of the failures either are directly related to anaesthetic care or at least occur in areas where obstetric anaesthetists have some influence.

BOX 5.7 Substandard care[6,9,14,20]

System failures
- High-risk women delivered in units without an on-site blood bank and/or intensive care unit.
- Consultant obstetricians and/or consultant anaesthetists not involved in high-risk cases.
- Poor communication between midwives, obstetricians and anaesthetists.

Failures in obstetric management
- Medical problems – pre-existing pregnancy not identified.
- Delay in diagnosis of ectopic pregnancy.
- Management plans not formulated for high-risk cases such as placenta praevia.
- Surgical misadventure.

Failures in the management of blood loss
- Failure to appreciate the severity of haemorrhage because cardiovascular system had not yet decompensated.
- Inadequate venous access.
- Underestimation of blood loss.
- Blood given too little and/or too late.
- Failure to warm transfused fluids.
- Over-transfusion of clear fluids.
- CVP and/or arterial line monitoring not used.
- Failure to diagnose and/or treat coagulopathy.

Management of major obstetric haemorrhage

Major obstetric haemorrhage has been defined in a number of different ways.[1,21] The author's preference is the definition used in his own hospital – that is, an estimated blood loss exceeding 1500 ml within 24 hours, or any substantial blood loss that causes significant deterioration in the patient's condition. Guidance on the management of major obstetric haemorrhage is given in Box 5.8. Some specific points are discussed in more detail below.

Hospital guidelines for major obstetric haemorrhage

Every maternity unit should have guidelines for the management of major obstetric haemorrhage, and should stage regular practice drills. Guidelines should cover organisational issues as well as guiding clinical management, and should be regularly reviewed.

Fluid and blood product replacement

Uterine blood flow at term is 700–900 ml/min, and the rate of blood loss during obstetric haemorrhage may be a significant proportion of this. In cases of severe haemorrhage, all fluids need to be given using a device that allows for rapid transfusion of warmed fluids sufficient to replace this rapid rate of loss. The objective should be to maintain blood pressure by maintaining normovolaemia. Under some circumstances (e.g. sepsis, acidosis) inotropes may need to be used, but they should not be a substitute for transfusing adequate volumes of fluid and red blood cells.

Guidance on fluid and blood product transfusion in cases of major obstetric haemorrhage is given in Box 5.9. Large volumes of clear fluids should be used with caution, as a number of haemorrhage deaths reported by the CEMD have been associated with over-transfusion of clear fluids. While a haemoglobin concentration as low as 7 g/dl may be acceptable in an obstetric patient who is neither actively bleeding nor anticipated to do so, transfusion of red blood cells should be commenced well above this level in cases of active bleeding. This is partly because it is easy to fall behind in transfusing blood if the haemorrhage becomes severe. In addition, when blood is first transfused the red blood cells have low levels of 2,3-diphosphoglycerate (2,3-DPG), causing a left shift in the oxygen dissociation curve. This significantly impairs the release of oxygen from haemoglobin into the tissues. The level of 2,3-DPG in transfused red blood cells returns to normal after 12–24 hours in the circulation.

The choice of additional blood components and the timing of their administration are complex.[25] Although there are various formulae which can be used, these are not strongly evidence based. Being guided by clotting studies may be inappropriate if the clinical situation is developing rapidly. Therefore a consultant haematologist should be involved early on in obstetric haemorrhage to give guidance on blood product replacement. Haematological involvement is essential if there is a coagulopathy.

The haematologist may suggest the use of recombinant factor VIIa (rFVIIa). This was originally developed to treat haemophiliacs, but has been used off licence to treat

BOX 5.8 Management of major obstetric haemorrhage[22–24]

General

- High-risk patients need an advance plan of management and should be delivered in a unit where blood bank and intensive care are available on site.
- When a major obstetric haemorrhage occurs, the hospital's guidelines for its clinical and organisational management should be automatically initiated.
- Senior surgical, anaesthetic and haematological help should be obtained.
- The measures listed below should be started in parallel, rather than performed in sequence.

Supportive measures

- Give the patient oxygen.
- If haemorrhage is antepartum, place the patient in a left lateral position.
- If the patient is hypotensive, place them in a head-down position.
- Insert at least two IV cannulas, minimum size 16 gauge.
- Take blood for a full blood count, clotting studies, crossmatching and electrolytes. Repeat after 4 units of red blood cells have been transfused (when fibrinogen should also be measured), and regularly thereafter.
- In the first instance, order 6 to 10 units of red blood cells.
- Restore normovolaemia with warm fluids and red blood cells (*see* Box 5.9).
- Insert a urinary catheter and attach a urimeter.
- Insert CVP and arterial lines (but this should not be allowed to delay further treatment).
- The patient should be kept warm by means of active warming devices.
- Consider the use of cell salvage.

Stopping the bleeding

- If appropriate, the baby and the placenta or placental fragments should be delivered.
- Management of uterine atony (which is often a component of the cause of obstetric haemorrhage) is covered in Box 5.4. Surgical intervention such as B-Lynch suture or hysterectomy may be required.
- Treat any coagulopathy with blood products (*see* Box 5.9).
- Consider radiological intervention.
- Consider giving antifibrinolytics.

Other measures

- If the baby is delivered, a paediatrician should be in attendance.
- Postoperative care should be in a high-dependency unit or an intensive-care unit, with involvement of an intensive-care specialist.
- Keep accurate contemporaneous records.

BOX 5.9 Fluid and blood product transfusion in major obstetric haemorrhage[23]

Clear fluids

- Red blood cells should be transfused as soon as possible. Until then, use:
  - crystalloid, maximum 2 litres
  - colloid, maximum 1.5 litres.
- Colloids, such as gelatin-containing fluids, remain initially almost entirely within the intravascular compartment, therefore restoring blood volume more quickly.

Red blood cells

- Depending on the urgency of the situation, give:
  - group O Rhesus D negative, 2 units should be immediately available
  - uncrossmatched ABO group specific, available quickly when blood group is known
  - fully crossmatched, usually is not available for at least half an hour.
- Monitor red blood cell replacement with regular haemoglobin estimation.

Fresh frozen plasma (FFP)

- Contains coagulation factors. Indications are as follows:
  - prothrombin time (PT) or activated partial thromboplastin time (APTT) is greater than 1.5 times normal, or
  - more than one blood volume has been replaced.
- Initial adult dose is 1 litre (4 units) or 15 ml/kg.
- Allow for 30 minutes' thawing time.

Platelets

- Likely to be required once 1.5 times blood volume has been replaced. Indications are as follows:
  - platelet count below 50×10^9/litre
  - platelet count below 100×10^9/litre with continuing serious bleeding.
- Initial adult dose is 250×10^9 (one pack of pooled platelets).
- May need to be obtained from a central blood transfusion centre.

Cryoprecipitate

- This contains fibrinogen and factor VIII. Indications are as follows:
  - fibrinogen level is less than 1 g/l, or
  - more than one blood volume has been replaced.
- Initial adult dose is 10 units.
- Early use of FFP may avoid the need for cryoprecipitate, as FFP also contains fibrinogen.

Recombinant factor VIIa and protein C

- May be appropriate in cases of severe coagulopathy. Discuss with the haematologist.

major haemorrhage. In a case report of 12 patients with postpartum haemorrhage who received rFVIIa, 11 patients responded well.[26] Likewise, some studies support the use of protein C if there is DIC.[18]

Anaesthesia for obstetric haemorrhage

Anaesthetic care for a major obstetric haemorrhage will need at least two or three anaesthetists and a similar number of anaesthetic support staff. A consultant anaesthetist should lead the team. Regional anaesthesia is contraindicated in major obstetric haemorrhage, as sympathetic blockade results in increased hypotension. The dose of induction agent for general anaesthesia may need to be reduced in patients who are hypovolaemic. It is probably better to use a familiar induction agent at a reduced dose than to use an unfamiliar agent. After induction of anaesthesia, care should be taken to avoid unnecessarily high concentrations of volatile anaesthetic agents, as these make uterine atony worse.

Monitoring

In addition to the standard for any anaesthetic, monitoring should also include a CVP line, an arterial line and urine output. A pulmonary artery catheter is not usually indicated.

Blood loss at delivery and during obstetric haemorrhage is difficult to assess and is frequently underestimated. Therefore CVP monitoring should be used if the cardiovascular system either is, or is likely to be, compromised by haemorrhage. The National Institute for Clinical Excellence (NICE) recommends considering the use of ultrasound guidance when CVP line insertion is necessary.[27] This is because its use is associated with a higher success rate and a lower incidence of complications. There is a case in the CEMD 1991–1993 report where there was difficulty inserting a CVP line using a landmark technique.[28] The patient had haemorrhaged after a Caesarean section, and had developed a coagulopathy. Following two failed attempts to insert an internal jugular CVP line, the patient developed a haematoma in her neck, which caused fatal airway obstruction. This is discussed further in Chapter 6.

An arterial line is essential in cases of major obstetric haemorrhage in order to assess blood pressure accurately, sample for blood gases, assess respiratory and acid–base status, and take samples to make haematological and biochemical measurements. Likewise, measurement of urine output is essential in order to monitor fluid balance and renal function.

Cell salvage

Cell salvage involves collecting blood from the operative field, separating out the red blood cells by centrifuge, and re-infusing them. No clotting factors or platelets are recovered. It is an option if the blood loss is intra-abdominal and is not heavily contaminated with amniotic fluid. NICE guidelines support its use in cases of obstetric haemorrhage, provided that a leukocyte depletion filter is used to reduce amniotic fluid contamination.[29] Cell salvage is of particular benefit to patients who refuse donated blood but accept salvaged blood. However, training is required to use a cell salvage machine, and its use will occupy an additional member of staff during the haemorrhage.

Risks of blood transfusion

The risks of blood transfusion, such as immunological reactions (e.g. ABO incompatibility) and infection (e.g. virus transmission) are well known. Massive blood transfusion brings additional problems, such as hypothermia and acute lung injury. Hypothermia may occur if fluids are inadequately warmed, and this may worsen coagulopathy. Metabolic problems such as hypocalcaemia and hyperkalaemia may also occur, and these are discussed below.

Very rapid blood transfusion used to be associated with hypocalcaemia due to the citrate anticoagulant that binds ionised calcium. However, the red cell preparations now available contain only traces of citrate. Fresh frozen plasma and platelet preparations do contain citrate, but are unlikely to be given in sufficient quantities to overwhelm the liver, which metabolises the citrate as part of the Krebs cycle. The exception is if the patient is hypothermic, as this slows citrate metabolism. This is another reason for maintaining normothermia, in addition to the deleterious effect of hypothermia on clotting. If there is ECG evidence of hypocalcaemia (i.e. a prolonged Q-T interval), the serum ionised calcium concentration may be below 1.0 mmol/l, and should be corrected with 5 ml of 10% calcium gluconate given by slow intravenous injection and repeated as required.

Hyperkalaemia can occur in massive blood transfusion as stored red blood cells release potassium into the solution in which they are suspended. A serum potassium concentration above 7 mmol/l may cause ventricular fibrillation, and this risk is increased by acidaemia and hypothermia. The ECG changes of hyperkalaemia are peaked T-waves, absent P-waves, widened QRS complexes and slurring of the S-T segment into T-waves. Treatment options include the physiological antagonist calcium, which can be given as described above. In addition, insulin with dextrose (10 units of insulin in 50 ml of 50% dextrose IV over 30–60 min) or salbutamol (50 µg bolus and 5–10 µg/min infusion IV) can be employed to increase cellular uptake of potassium.

Stored red blood cells do reabsorb potassium once they have been transfused, and this sometimes results in subsequent hypokalaemia. The ECG changes of hypokalaemia are S-T segment depression, Q-T and P-R interval prolongation, T-wave inversion and appearance of a U-wave. Treatment is with dilute IV potassium chloride transfused at up to 40 mmol/hour. ECG monitoring is required, as too rapid administration may cause hyperkalaemia and ventricular fibrillation.

Antifibrinolytics

There is some evidence to support the use of tranexamic acid and aprotinin in obstetric haemorrhage.[30-33] Both work by inhibiting the breakdown of fibrin. However, they may worsen the effects of DIC, and they also increase the risk of thromboembolic phenomena. Tranexamic acid is both cheaper and less likely to cause allergic reactions than aprotinin, and is recommended in the CEMD guidelines for haemorrhage in women who refuse blood transfusions (*see* Box 5.5).

B-Lynch suture and radiological intervention

The CEMD 1997–1999 and 2000–2002 reports advocate the use of both of these techniques. The B-Lynch suture has been previously discussed in the section on uterine atony. Like the B-Lynch suture, radiological embolisation is becoming increasingly popular for controlling obstetric haemorrhage. Embolisation is only a possibility if the patient is sufficiently stable to allow transfer to the radiology department. However, bilateral iliac artery balloon catheters can be inserted under portable image-intensifier control within the obstetric theatre. No deaths have been reported to the CEMD in cases where a B-Lynch suture has been used, and only one death has been reported where radiological embolisation was employed. Both of these techniques warrant further scientific evaluation.

Conclusion

Although there are many different types of obstetric haemorrhage, the principles of its management are always the same.

- The likelihood of haemorrhage in high-risk patients should be anticipated.
- There should be a low threshold for diagnosing significant haemorrhage, even if the patient shows little sign of physiological compromise.
- Surgical and anaesthetic management should be undertaken by senior staff.
- Early liaison with haematologists is needed, with prompt replacement of red blood cells and other blood products.

If these principles are followed, even more mothers will survive obstetric haemorrhage.

CHAPTER 6

Hypertension

MICHAEL KINSELLA AND MARK SCRUTTON

Pre-eclampsia is a disease specific to human pregnancy, although some inexact animal models have been used to investigate the pathophysiology. It is in some way immunologically mediated, and may develop because the immune barriers in the placenta have been sacrificed in order to allow for the long human pregnancy and the development of the relatively large newborn. The trophoblast fails to invade the spiral arteries of the myometrium, a process that normally leads to their extensive enlargement and reduction in flow resistance.[1] The systemic cardiovascular changes of pregnancy are impaired so that a pre-eclamptic woman's responses to catecholamines, for instance, are not reduced as in the normal pregnant circulation, but remain the same as in the non-pregnant circulation.[2] Systemic endothelial changes develop that may affect multiple organs, with the lungs, liver and brain being especially sensitive.[3] The placenta becomes compromised, causing intra-uterine growth restriction of the fetus. The effects are variable. Some women present with largely fetal compromise, some with largely maternal compromise and some with both.[3] Maternal cerebral, haematological or hepatic dysfunction may present before the classic combination of hypertension and proteinuria, and the speed of deterioration is unpredictable.

CEMD 2000–2002 report[4]

The 2000–2002 report focuses on early diagnosis and rapid effective treatment of pre-eclampsia guided by local protocols directly managed by consultant obstetricians, obstetric anaesthetists and intensive-care specialists. Maternity units require guidelines for the initial and ongoing management of severe pre-eclampsia. There is now considerable evidence available to guide the development of management protocols. An annex to the hypertension chapter of the 1997–1999 report included pre-eclampsia management guidelines from the Mersey Region.[5] To prevent delays and inconsistencies in treatment, many regions have moved to standardised treatment pathways (*see* Box 6.1). Initial treatment of hypertension with oral labetalol (first-line therapy) or oral nifedipine (second-line therapy) allows immediate delivery of the drug to the patient. Hydralazine was a more popular first-line agent in the past, but

---

BOX 6.1 Protocol for the treatment of hypertension in severe pre-eclampsia

First-line agent: labetalol
200 mg orally (repeat after 30 minutes)
OR
50 mg IV bolus (repeat every 5 minutes up to a maximum dose of 200 mg)
followed by 20–160 mg/hour IV infusion
Note: Contraindicated in asthma.

Second-line agent: nifedipine
10 mg orally (repeat after 30 minutes)

Third-line agent: hydralazine
5 mg IV over 15 minutes (repeat after 30 minutes)
followed by 2–8 mg/hour IV infusion

---

had to be given by multiple intravenous injections that needed to be administered by a doctor. Consultant obstetricians should be involved early on in order to ensure prompt intervention. Severe hypertension, particularly systolic hypertension, needs to be defined in local guidelines and treated effectively. In deteriorating situations, intensive-care specialists should be involved in a timely manner.

Initial diagnosis of pre-eclampsia is often missed or delayed. Pregnant women presenting with headache or new epigastric pain require blood pressure measurement and urinalysis to exclude pre-eclampsia. Automated non-invasive blood pressure monitors may underestimate blood pressure to a significant degree, and therefore conventional sphygmomanometers should be used for confirmation.[6] In the presence of significant organ dysfunction but unremarkable hypertension, severe hypertension may occur rapidly and unexpectedly, but must be identified and treated as early as possible.

TABLE 6.1 Number of deaths by cause due to eclampsia and pre-eclampsia, for the period 1985–2002, in the UK

CAUSE	1985–87	1988–90	1991–93	1994–96	1997–99	2000–02
Cerebral	11	14	5	7	7	9
Pulmonary	11	10	11	8	2	1
Other	5	3	4	5	7	4
Total	27	27	20	20	16	14

Pulmonary complications of pre-eclampsia, in particular those caused by pulmonary oedema and fluid overload, have become a less frequent cause of maternal death since 1997 (*see* Table 6.1). However, fluid balance must be carefully monitored and restricted. Central venous pressure monitoring should be considered early on.

Medical (obstetric) management
Hypertension

CASE 1 (1997–1999)[5]

A woman was admitted to hospital with what appeared to be mild pre-eclampsia, and planned induction of labour was delayed because the delivery suite was busy. In the meantime, she developed fulminating pre-eclampsia accompanied by epigastric pain and unusual patterns of behaviour, and she received treatment with hydralazine but no anticonvulsant. Two hours later, she had an eclamptic fit, which was treated with intravenous diazepam and phenytoin infusion. Some hours after delivery by Caesarean section, she became drowsy and developed focal neurological signs. She had suffered an intracranial haemorrhage and was transferred to a regional neurosurgical unit where she underwent three craniotomies, but to no avail. A previously undiagnosed arteriovenous malformation was found at the site of haemorrhage.

Intracranial haemorrhage remains the leading cause of death in pre-eclampsia and eclampsia. The absolute number of maternal deaths from this complication remains unchanged since 1985 (*see* Table 6.1). It usually occurs in women with no underlying cerebral pathology at levels of blood pressure that would not normally be a significant risk in an otherwise healthy individual. The other pathological processes occurring in pre-eclampsia, such as endothelial damage in blood vessels, decreased blood coagulability and changes in regional cerebral blood flow, contribute significantly to the risk of haemorrhage. However, hypertension is the most readily treatable of these factors, and the importance of its urgent and effective treatment is emphasised in the CEMD 2000–2002 report.[4]

In Case 1, an unsuspected arteriovenous malformation was discovered. The 1997–1999 and 2000–2002 reports concluded that bleeding from a cerebral aneurysm or arteriovenous malformation in non-pre-eclamptic women is unlikely to be related to labour, and the effect of pregnancy in itself is unclear, given that aneurysms often bleed during the postpartum period.[4,5] As such pathology is often unknown, the only way in which these events can be prevented is by tight blood pressure control in all cases of pre-eclampsia.

Significance of systolic and mean blood pressure
Pre-eclampsia is associated with blood pressure values of ≥ 140/90 mmHg. Severe pre-eclampsia is usually defined by a blood pressure of > 160/110 mmHg or a

mean blood pressure of 125 mmHg. In the past, treatment of chronic hypertension outside pregnancy focused on controlling diastolic blood pressure, and this was the same with the treatment of raised blood pressure in pre-eclampsia. The rationale is that elevation of diastolic blood pressure reflects an increase in arteriolar tone and systemic vascular resistance. The pulse pressure (the difference between systolic and diastolic pressure) is increased by two factors. These are increased stroke volume, related to a hyperdynamic circulation, and increased stiffness of the large arteries, although the latter effect is less relevant in the pregnant population. More recently, however, it has become clear that the importance of systolic hypertension in both pregnant and non-pregnant populations has been overlooked.

Some pre-eclampsia guidelines suggest the use of mean arterial pressure. This is done automatically with electronic blood pressure measurement methods, but has to be calculated if using sphygmomanometry. The mean blood pressure reflects both systolic and diastolic components of blood pressure. The CEMD 2000–2002 report states:

> It is thought to be the pressure during systole which causes intracerebral haemorrhage. Recognition of this concept should be incorporated into clinical guidelines to try to ensure effective reduction of systolic pressure. It is, therefore, recommended that clinical protocols identify a systolic blood pressure above which urgent and effective antihypertensive treatment is required. Some would recommend 160 mmHg as a useful guide to treatment. Consideration should also be given to starting early antihypertensive treatment when the blood pressure is not, in itself, alarming but where the severity of the pre-eclampsia makes a rapid increase in pressure likely.[4]

CASE 2 (2000–2002)[4]

This patient, whose blood pressure was 110/60 mmHg in early pregnancy, was admitted in late pregnancy with a diastolic pressure of 92 mmHg and proteinuria (+++). Over the subsequent days, blood pressures of 155/95 mmHg and 145/100 mmHg were noted. Induction of labour was delayed due to a lack of special care baby unit cots. The woman's blood pressure was 160/105 mmHg and there was proteinuria (++++). The following day, she complained of epigastric pain and a puffy face. Her blood pressure was 170/105 mmHg. Attempts were made to induce labour despite an unfavourable cervix. After her blood pressure rose to 220/120 mmHg, antihypertensive treatment was started for the first time (intravenous labetalol). Her blood pressure remained elevated at 215/120 mmHg and she remained symptomatic. A Caesarean section was performed. There was continuing poor control of the patient's blood pressure after delivery. She developed twitching, slurred speech and mouth dropping, and was seen for the first time since admission by a consultant obstetrician. A computed tomography (CT) scan showed a massive intracranial haemorrhage.

In this case, it is notable that along with grossly elevated systolic blood pressure, diastolic blood pressure was not treated until it reached 120 mmHg, and even then not effectively. Although it may be argued that effective treatment of diastolic blood pressure is likely to simultaneously control systolic blood pressure, a key issue is to make sure that systolic hypertension is not overlooked. Finally, while absolute values of both systolic and diastolic pressures are important, any significant increase from the woman's normal non-pregnant blood pressure, sometimes best judged by the 'booking' blood pressure in early pregnancy, must be taken into account.

CASE 3 (1997–1999)[5]

A woman with a multiple pregnancy had a blood pressure at booking of 90/60 mmHg. She was admitted to hospital during the pregnancy with pre-eclampsia, and was subsequently delivered by Caesarean section. Immediately prior to delivery, her blood pressure was 140/80 mmHg and she had proteinuria (+++). There was inadequate monitoring of the patient's blood pressure after delivery, but the pressure was found to be 260/140 mmHg some 8 hours after the birth. The patient developed neurological symptoms and was transferred to the ICU, where it became obvious that she had suffered a cerebral haemorrhage. Autopsy revealed a pontine haemorrhage.

In this case, postoperative monitoring of the patient's blood pressure was substandard, as was the failure to provide prompt and effective treatment of a rise in blood pressure greatly in excess of baseline levels.

Significance of the method used to measure blood pressure

The last two CEMD reports, for 1997–1999 and 2000–2002, highlighted the pitfalls of using automated non-invasive blood pressure (NIBP) devices.[4,5] These allow regular blood pressure measurements without taking up midwifery time, and they display heart rate and mean blood pressure. Concerns about health hazards associated with mercury have led to withdrawal of the mercury-column sphygmomanometer, but aneroid sphygmomanometers are prone to significant error unless calibration is rigorously checked. Although automated NIBP devices may be used for most readings, the results must be compared periodically with manual measurement in order to rule out significant inaccuracies.[6]

The 1997–1999 report[5] stated:

> Another important point to note is the potential for misleading blood pressure measurements from automated recording systems, which can systematically underestimate both systolic and diastolic blood pressures in pre-eclampsia to an alarming degree.[6] These systems are useful to monitor trends during treatment, but the values should be compared, at the beginning, with those obtained by conventional sphygmomanometers. It is critically important in ensuring that life-

threatening, severe hypertension is treated effectively, that the blood pressure is measured accurately, otherwise the degree of hypertension may be underestimated. In a woman with severe disease there may be merit in the insertion of an arterial line to measure blood pressure.

The 2000–2002 Report[4] reiterated this:

> It is also worth re-emphasising, as in the last Report, the observation that many automated blood pressure monitoring systems systematically underestimate systolic pressure in pre-eclampsia. Mercury sphygmomanometers should be used to establish baseline blood pressure as a reference for automated monitoring in hospital for women with pre-eclampsia, unless the automated system has been validated in pregnancy.[7]

Severe hypertension may be an indication to use intra-arterial blood pressure (IABP) measurement. Although high blood pressure may cause direct vascular damage, excessively rapid blood pressure reduction that outstrips the decrease in vascular resistance may lead to reduced blood flow in the brain, heart, placenta and kidneys. If rapid maternal stabilisation requiring intravenous antihypertensive treatment is needed, the use of IABP should be strongly considered (*see* Box 6.2).

It is not practicable to perform frequent (at 1-minute intervals) NIBP readings for a prolonged time, so IABP may also be required in situations where rapid fluctuations of blood pressure are anticipated, such as during active or second-stage labour and anaesthetic induction and reversal (*see* Box 6.2).

Drug treatment for control of hypertension

CASE 4 (1988–1990)[8]

A multigravida at 26 weeks' gestation was found to have a blood pressure of 160/100 mmHg with marked proteinuria (++). She was admitted and an SHO prescribed an oral slow-release calcium-channel-blocking agent. Overnight the diastolic blood pressure was in the range 105–120 mmHg, and the patient was prescribed anti-emetics for nausea and vomiting. Control of oral medication was difficult because of persistent vomiting. The same oral antihypertensive drug was repeated the following morning when the patient was seen by a different team. As the diastolic blood pressure was still in the range 100–130 mmHg, it was suggested that she should be seen by the consultant in the afternoon. When she was eventually seen by the consultant 22 hours after admission, she was transferred to a high-dependency area and given a bolus of hydralazine intravenously followed by further oral antihypertensive therapy. Her blood pressure then fell steeply to 130/75 mmHg, but the proteinuria increased. The following morning the patient was found unconscious, and she died soon afterwards. Autopsy showed brainstem infarction, hypertensive encephalopathy and the renal changes of severe pre-eclampsia.

BOX 6.2 Indications for invasive cardiovascular access in pre-eclampsia

Arterial

Pressure monitoring – beat-by-beat values required
- Blood pressure changes occur in less than 1 minute.
- Labour with persisting hypertension.
- Induction of anaesthesia for Caesarean section, poorly controlled blood pressure.
- Tracheal extubation, poorly controlled blood pressure.

Pressure monitoring – difficulties with non-invasive blood pressure measurement
- Haemorrhage.
- Obesity.
- HDU care – frequent blood pressure measurements required.
- HDU care – proven discrepancy between automatic non-invasive blood pressure and sphygmomanometer measurements.

Other factors
- Repeated arterial blood gas sampling if there are problems with oxygenation.
- Frequent blood sampling.

Central venous pressure

Pressure monitoring
- Haemorrhage.
- Coagulopathy, HELLP.
- Persisting oliguria.
- Suspicion of myocardial dysfunction, pulmonary problems.
- Delayed delivery and significant fluid infusion.

Other factors
- Poor peripheral venous access.
- Frequent blood sampling.
- Irritant or vasoactive drug infusions.

Hypertension must be controlled urgently and effectively before delivery whenever possible. Delivery will start the resolution of pre-eclampsia, but performing an emergency Caesarean section while blood pressure remains uncontrolled increases morbidity and mortality. In exceptional circumstances, delivery may be required before full stabilisation has occurred – for example, in cases of severe fetal compromise. However, this puts the mother at greater risk and therefore must be carefully considered. In most cases, including eclampsia, the patient should be monitored, investigated and stabilised before delivery. Blood pressure must be controlled effectively but not reduced excessively quickly, for the reasons outlined above. Thus the process of stabilisation may take 2 to 4 hours.

In mild to moderate hypertension during pregnancy, blood pressure control may be managed either in the community or as an inpatient while trying to prolong the pregnancy to allow fetal maturation. In these settings, methyldopa remains the cornerstone of antihypertensive therapy, due to its well-established safety record, particularly the lack of fetal complications. Outside pregnancy, methyldopa is rarely used to treat hypertension, as newer agents are more effective and have better side-effect profiles, but some remain untested in pregnancy and others are recognised as having potentially serious fetal side-effects. For example, angiotensin-converting enzyme (ACE) inhibitors cause fetal renal impairment and oligohydramnios. Nonetheless, as experience with newer drugs increases, it is likely that methyldopa may eventually be superseded.

In severe hypertension, traditionally and intuitively rapid control of blood pressure would seem to require the use of intravenous agents. In the UK, hydralazine was frequently chosen as the first-line agent. However, a meta-analysis published in 2003 suggested that maternal and fetal side-effects were worse with hydralazine, such that its use as a first-line agent could not be supported.[9] This may be because of an excessively rapid reduction in blood pressure. Furthermore, intravenous drugs require intravenous access, careful preparation, and complex administration (by syringe pumps) under senior guidance and careful monitoring. This may result in a significant delay in drug delivery and an increase in the likelihood of error, particularly overdose.

Subsequent to this meta-analysis,[9] many units have adopted labetalol or nifedipine as first-line agents. Oral administration is simple, rapid and unlikely to result in a catastrophic reduction in blood pressure, so long as the sublingual route is avoided if nifedipine is used (*see* Box 6.1). However, the intravenous route is necessary if enteral absorption is unreliable, as in Case 4.

CASE 5 (1988–1990)[8]

A primigravida at 29 weeks' gestation had a blood pressure of 140/110 mmHg and proteinuria (++++). Labour was induced with vaginal prostaglandins. The blood pressure was poorly controlled in labour, which lasted 10 hours, during which the patient had an eclamptic fit. In the course of this she vomited and aspirated. It had been hoped that an epidural would control her blood pressure. She received no other form of antihypertensive therapy in labour before the fit.

Epidural analgesia in labour relieves pain and reduces blood catecholamine levels.[10] The former leads to a reduction in blood pressure towards the baseline value found before labour, and attenuates the increases in blood pressure during active contractions. These effects may be sufficient to avoid the need for other antihypertensive medication, and if an epidural is intended, it may be sensible to

> **BOX 6.3** Protocol for administration of magnesium sulphate in severe pre-eclampsia and eclampsia[6,10]
>
> | | |
> |---|---|
> | Loading dose: | 4 g IV over 15–20 minutes |
> | Maintenance dose: | 1 g/hour IV infusion |
> | Further fits: | 2 g over 5–10 minutes |
>
> **Indications to consider laboratory measurement of serum magnesium levels**
> - Infusion for longer than 36 hours.
> - Repeat boluses for recurrent fits.
> - Oliguria.
> - Clinical: hyporeflexia, weakness, respiratory depression, cardiac dysrhythmia.

establish this before starting specific medication. However, the extent of blood pressure reduction is not predictable in individual cases, and an epidural should never take the place of specific antihypertensive medication.

Eclampsia

Eclampsia and magnesium prophylaxis

The results of the Collaborative Eclampsia Trial in 1995 represent the most dramatic example of evidence-based medicine leading to a significant change in clinical practice, with the use of magnesium in eclampsia in the UK increasing from 2% in 1992 to 90% in 2001.[11–13] The exact mechanism of action of magnesium as an anticonvulsant in eclampsia remains uncertain. However, focal cerebral ischaemia is a feature of severe pre-eclampsia,[14] and magnesium may reverse this, as it is known to produce cerebral vasodilation. It is not relevant to comment on anticonvulsant regimens from the earlier reports, but by 1997–1999 (Case 1)[5] it was considered substandard care not to use a magnesium infusion after a convulsion (*see* Box 6.3).[11]

During 2000–2002, two women died after receiving magnesium sulphate for presumed eclampsia, but they were subsequently found to have other pathology, primary cerebral haemorrhage and bacterial meningitis.[4] In a woman who does not have epilepsy, the most likely cause of a convulsion in the second or third trimester is eclampsia, and the safety profile of magnesium is such as to warrant immediate treatment for this presumptive diagnosis. However, if the clinical picture does not match fully, an open mind should always be kept to the possibility of other pathology.

Choice of drug for treatment for convulsions

Eclamptic convulsions are self-limiting, lasting on average 90 seconds. Although diazepam has been advocated in the past to treat the convulsion itself, current opinion suggests that magnesium is more appropriate.[15] A prolonged fit may prompt consideration of diazepam or thiopentone, but should also suggest an alternative diagnosis as stated above. The latter drugs may cause significant ventilatory and cardiovascular depression and prolong the period of risk of pulmonary aspiration of stomach contents. The Collaborative Eclampsia Trial found that magnesium was the most effective treatment for preventing recurrent convulsions in eclampsia, but 11% of women in total were given magnesium and 64% were given other anticonvulsants before starting the allocated trial medication.[11] The effectiveness of magnesium for the treatment of a convulsion has never been assessed.

Threshold for magnesium prophylaxis in pre-eclampsia

CASE 6 (1997–1999)[5]

This patient had a blood pressure of 100/60 mmHg at booking. She developed vomiting and diarrhoea in mid third trimester. On arrival at hospital, she was found to have a blood pressure of 210/120 mmHg with proteinuria (++++). There was difficulty in contacting the on-call consultant, and 1 hour after admission and before any treatment had been given the patient had an eclamptic fit. She was treated with magnesium sulphate and labetalol and delivered by Caesarean section. Continuing management was discussed with the consultant in charge of the local ICU, which was on another site, and the decision was made to continue the patient's care in the high-dependency unit in the maternity unit. Despite further treatment with labetalol and hydralazine, the patient remained hypertensive, and she had a cardiac arrest 4 hours after delivery. She was resuscitated and transferred to the ICU, but a CT scan revealed a massive intracranial haemorrhage.

The CEMD 1997–1999 report concluded that in this case the delay in administering antihypertensive medication was more important than the delay in giving the anticonvulsant.[5] Subsequently, in 2002, the findings of the Magpie Trial were published, establishing the effectiveness of magnesium in reducing the likelihood of developing eclampsia.[15] This trial found that the number needed to treat in order to prevent eclampsia was 63 in severe pre-eclampsia and 109 for women without severe pre-eclampsia. In today's practice, it is likely that the woman in Case 6 with severe pre-eclampsia might have been given magnesium prophylaxis. However, due to lack of clear evidence, clinicians remain inconsistent in defining the threshold of severity of pre-eclampsia at which magnesium prophylaxis should be started.

Aspiration

From the second trimester of pregnancy onwards, women are considered to be at risk of pulmonary aspiration during periods of unconsciousness, due to reduced lower oesophageal tone and increased intragastric pressure. During labour, stomach emptying is delayed, especially if opioids are given. The earlier CEMD reports recognise aspiration as a complication both of prolonged convulsions and of the old anticonvulsant regimens.

CASE 7 (1985–1987)[16]

A parous woman was noted by her general practitioner to have a trace of proteinuria, and a blood pressure of 130/84 mmHg. No action was taken, and several days later she had an eclamptic fit. Her general practitioner did not visit her, but arranged for her admission to a hospital half a mile away from the obstetric unit. She was taken unsedated to a medical unit, and had two fits en route. A junior obstetric staff member made a diagnosis of a neurological condition and sent her to the medical intensive-therapy unit. She was over-sedated with drugs that are rarely used in obstetric practice, and grossly overloaded with intravenous fluids. She delivered a stillborn baby and died 48 hours after admission from cardiovascular failure due to eclampsia, complicated by aspiration of vomit.

Aspiration has only rarely been highlighted as a complication of eclampsia in recent triennia. It possibly occurred in a woman who died from adult respiratory distress syndrome (ARDS) after a convulsion in 1985–1987, and in 1994–1996 a woman died from ARDS precipitated by Mendelson's syndrome after aspiration during an eclamptic fit at home.[16,17] We speculate that this reduction in aspiration has resulted from a decrease in the use of diazepam and greater emphasis on keeping the stomach empty. Women who are given magnesium or who are considered to be at risk of losing consciousness from other causes should have the same nil-by-mouth and antacid regimen as those who are considered to be likely to require general anaesthesia (*see* Chapter 3).

Haemolysis, elevated liver enzymes, low platelets (HELLP) syndrome
Coagulopathy and platelets
Several cases from the CEMD 1997–1999 report describe severe HELLP syndrome.

CASE 8 (1997–1999)[5]

This patient was admitted to hospital in late pregnancy with what appeared to be mild pre-eclampsia. Her blood pressure was modestly elevated at 150/90 mmHg, there was proteinuria (++++), and her uric acid levels and platelet counts were normal. Induction of labour was started, but the patient complained of severe abdominal pain and became markedly hypertensive.

She was treated with labetalol and magnesium sulphate and delivered by Caesarean section. It was apparent that she had HELLP syndrome, with falling haemoglobin concentration and platelet counts and rapidly rising liver function test results. There was also deteriorating renal function. A decision was made to transfer the patient to an ICU (the maternity unit was isolated) after she became drowsy some 6 hours after delivery. On arrival at the ICU, she was found to have pulmonary oedema. She did not have a central line. There was also evidence of intracranial haemorrhage, which ultimately was responsible for her death. Autopsy revealed subdural blood and a large intracerebral haematoma, as well as liver necrosis.

CASE 9 (1997–1999)[5]

A very young woman was admitted to hospital early in the third trimester because her fetus was small for gestational age and there had been reduced fetal movement. Steroids were given. The blood pressure was normal on admission, and biochemistry was also normal except for a marginally raised uric acid level. Three days later the patient complained of visual disturbance and abdominal pain, and the next day was noted to have elevated blood pressure, proteinuria, hyper-reflexia and grossly disordered biochemical and haematological results compatible with HELLP syndrome. Delivery was undertaken by Caesarean section, but the fulminating pattern of disease continued, requiring treatment with magnesium sulphate (which was subsequently stopped because of oliguria), haematological input, and transfer to the ICU some 16 hours after delivery. Ventilation was commenced in the ICU, but the woman remained gravely ill and she died 4 days later. Autopsy confirmed the presence of multi-organ damage, including ARDS, acute tubular necrosis, liver changes typical of severe pre-eclampsia/HELLP syndrome, pituitary infarction and hypoxic changes in the brain.

Coagulopathy can develop suddenly and precipitously both before and after delivery, and deterioration may occur over 24 hours after delivery. HELLP is not easy to diagnose, and there must be a low threshold of suspicion leading to regular biochemical testing. There may be a reluctance to institute central venous monitoring in the face of coagulopathy, particularly when patients are outside the ICU being cared for by clinicians who are less familiar with the use of invasive monitoring. Obstetric anaesthetists must be prepared to place central lines readily in such circumstances, if necessary considering the correction of coagulopathy with administration of blood products and the use of ultrasound guidance to minimise the risk of complications. Obstetric anaesthetists with few ICU skills must recognise the need for immediate involvement of their ICU colleagues.

Liver haematoma and rupture

Upper abdominal pain in pregnancy, particularly if it is on the right side, must be treated with a high index of suspicion, as it may be an early sign of liver swelling.[18]

As has been mentioned previously, a combination of increased distending pressure from hypertension, endothelial damage in blood vessels and decreased blood coagulability represents prime risk factors for bleeding complications. In this situation, inflammation of the liver leads to swelling, with the potential for subcapsular haematoma.

CASE 10 (1994–1996)[17]

Delay in delivery also occurred, due to efforts to gain fetal maturity. This patient was admitted at 28 weeks' gestation, complaining of upper abdominal pain which was unrelieved by antacid. She had hypertension and proteinuria (+++). She was admitted to hospital and steroids were initiated to enhance fetal lung maturity. Three days after admission, the patient complained of backache, epigastric pain and nausea. Her blood pressure was subsequently recorded as 200/120 mmHg. She was found in a post-ictal state. She was stabilised and transferred by ambulance to the regional perinatal centre, which was 10 minutes away. Intrauterine fetal death occurred, labour was induced and uncontrollable intraperitoneal haemorrhage occurred. At laparotomy, subcapsular haematoma and liver rupture were found to be present, and the results of liver function tests taken earlier that day showed grossly elevated liver enzymes.

CASE 11 (1997–1999)[5]

A parous woman with pre-eclampsia was admitted to hospital. Her blood pressure was modestly elevated. She was allowed home, but returned later the same day after the GP was called and found her blood pressure to be 220/120 mmHg. In hospital, her blood pressure was 160/120 mmHg and she complained of epigastric pain. She had proteinuria (+++), haematuria, thrombocytopenia and brisk reflexes. Urgent delivery by Caesarean section was planned, but was delayed somewhat because of another acute problem in the hospital. In the meantime, the patient became shocked and the fetal heart stopped. At Caesarean section, a major haemoperitoneum was found, arising from a ruptured subcapsular haematoma of the liver. There was also a major postpartum uterine haemorrhage requiring hysterectomy. The patient was transferred to another hospital and underwent partial hepatectomy. She was considered for liver transplantation, but her poor clinical state made this option non-viable [by the time a donor organ was available].

This case illustrates the risk of major haemorrhage from the liver. The clinical course is likely to be overwhelming, irrespective of the quality of medical care.

Pulmonary damage

The CEMD 1985–1987 report[16] first drew attention to an increase in pulmonary causes of death (*see* Table 6.1):

> There has been a striking increase in this triennium in the number of deaths from pulmonary complications, which were the immediate cause of death in 12 out of the 27 deaths. This is the first time that the occurrence of ARDS in patients dying from a hypertensive disorder has been noted in these reports. There were nine deaths from this cause, and this occurred 4 to 21 (average 13) days after delivery. It is possible that patients who might previously have died at an earlier stage from severe cerebral complications are now, as a result of modern techniques of resuscitation, living long enough to develop changes in the lungs, perhaps aggravated by fluid imbalance, leading to interference with exchange of blood gases and eventually death from hypoxia and multi-organ failure.

Fluid flux in the lung

The Starling equation determines the rate of fluid transfer from the blood to the pulmonary interstitial fluid:

$$\text{Fluid flux} = K \left[(P_c - P_i) - r \left(\pi_c - \pi_i \right) \right]$$

where K = filtration coefficient, r = reflection coefficient, P = hydrostatic pressure, π = colloid oncotic pressure, and the suffixes c and i refer to capillary and interstitial pressure, respectively.

Factors that increase the hydrostatic pressure gradient or reduce the colloid oncotic pressure (COP) gradient will increase the rate of flux. The plasma COP is determined by the protein concentration. An increase in interstitial COP may occur if there is an increase in permeability to proteins (a reduction in the reflection coefficient) following damage to the pulmonary capillary membrane. In this situation, the hydrostatic pressure gradient becomes critical. The hydrostatic pressure gradient can be minimised by reducing the pulmonary capillary wedge pressure (PCWP), or by applying positive airway pressure to the alveoli.

The Starling equation is often simplified to a clinically usable measure of the safety margin for fluid transfer, the COP–PCWP gradient. This gradient is reduced by various salient physiological factors, namely pregnancy, delivery reaching the lowest point at 6 hours, and pre-eclampsia.[19,20] The normal non-pregnant value for COP is 25–28 mmHg, but in pre-eclampsia it may be halved to 14 mmHg.[20] Intravenous fluid prehydration of 20 ml/kg reduced the COP significantly more than 10 ml/kg, although 30 ml/kg did not increase this effect further.[21] In a study of 10 pre-eclamptic women who developed pulmonary oedema, three had ARDS due to pulmonary damage, two had left ventricular failure, and five had a reduced COP–PCWP gradient.[22]

Fluid overload

CASE 12 (1994–1996)[17]

This patient, apparently due to fear of hospitals, failed to attend for antenatal care, and presented in labour at 37 weeks' gestation with severe iron-deficiency anaemia and severe pre-eclampsia (+++ proteinuria and a blood pressure of 180/100 mmHg). She also had a microcytic anaemia with a haemoglobin level of 5 g/dl. Four units of blood were transfused rapidly, the baby was delivered by ventouse, blood pressure was controlled with hydralazine and phenytoin was given. The patient developed severe pulmonary oedema, was transferred to the ICU, subsequently developed ARDS and died 1 month after delivery from complications of ARDS.

This case demonstrated pulmonary oedema secondary to inappropriate rapid transfusion in a normovolaemic woman. Blood is retained in the circulation for a prolonged period, and will lead to a marked and sustained increase in pulmonary capillary hydrostatic pressure.

More common is over-transfusion of crystalloid or colloid, as in Case 8 and the following examples.

CASE 13 (2000–2002)[4]

This patient was admitted to hospital in late second trimester with pre-eclampsia. Her first pregnancy had been complicated by early severe pre-eclampsia, and the second pregnancy was normal. Her blood pressure was only modestly elevated, but she had proteinuria (++++). A decision was made to deliver her the next day by Caesarean section after administration of corticosteroids. That night, she had a placental abruption and was delivered by Caesarean section. Postoperatively, she received a massive intravenous fluid overload without any central monitoring. She subsequently died in the intensive-care unit, from a combination of ARDS and pneumonia.

CASE 14 (1988–1990)[8]

This patient, who had raised blood pressure, proteinuria and fetal growth retardation, was admitted at 35 weeks' gestation and had a fit 2 hours after admission, before any urine testing or careful observation of blood pressure had been undertaken. Caesarean section was performed the same evening, but overnight her care was substandard. Extra fluid was given postpartum to 'chase a low urine output', and a CVP line was said to be 'not working.' The following morning the patient was transferred to an ICU, where she died 10 days later from ARDS.

A key goal of ICU treatment in the 1980s was to administer fluids and inotropes in order to produce supranormal levels of cardiac output and oxygen delivery.[23] Evidence of intravascular volume depletion in some cases of pre-eclampsia reinforced the liberal administration of both crystalloid and colloid. The COP–PCWP gradient is evidently worsened by crystalloid, and some centres have therefore favoured colloid use. However, in pre-eclampsia, colloids will pass across malfunctioning capillary membranes into the pulmonary interstitium, reducing the transcapillary oncotic gradient. Pulmonary oedema may be reversible, but if there is any further damage to the pulmonary capillary membrane, ARDS may occur with an associated high mortality.

A temporary oliguria after delivery secondary to intrinsic renal mechanisms and secretion of pituitary hormones is normal, and is more pronounced in pre-eclampsia. Since the mid-1990s, unmonitored and aggressive expansion of plasma volume in order to produce a diuresis has become uncommon.

The CEMD 1994–1996 report noted that intravenous fluid overload sometimes occurred because the obstetrician, anaesthetist and haematologist prescribed fluids independently, and the report suggested that one member of staff should hold responsibility for overall fluid management.[17] If a 'maintenance fluid' regimen of 80 ml/hour is prescribed, other infusions such as Syntocinon, magnesium and glucose/insulin infusions must be included in the total. These infusions can be given through a syringe pump in a concentrated form, rather than by volumetric infusion. Furthermore, oral fluids are preferable to intravenous maintenance fluid when gut function is normal.[24]

Central venous pressure (CVP) monitoring

There are limited indications for invasive monitoring of CVP if simple intravenous fluid overload, as in Cases 8 and 14, is avoided. Significant blood loss and blood transfusion, as in Cases 12 and 13, would be indications for central venous catheter (CVC) insertion (*see* Box 6.2) in non-obstetric cases, although there is sometimes a reluctance to use invasive monitoring on the labour ward (highlighted in the anaesthetic section of several CEMD reports up to 2000–2002). Because of the disease process, a hypovolaemic woman with pre-eclampsia may be apparently 'normotensive.'

CVC placement may also be required if there are concerns about persisting oliguria, initially to exclude subnormal CVP implying hypovolaemia, and then to ensure that, if given, fluid challenge does not increase CVP above normal. Fluids should not be administered in order to elevate the CVP to an arbitrary target value.

CASE 15 (1991–1993)[25]

A woman with sickle-cell trait and a history of a previous Caesarean section required emergency Caesarean section due to worsening pre-eclampsia. The anaesthetist, who was a registrar, reported no problems. After surgery, a Syntocinon infusion was set up because of a poorly contracted uterus, and the patient was transferred to the high-dependency area. There was continuing blood loss and coagulopathy. Exploration under general anaesthesia found the bleeding to be from the wound itself. An hour later there was very little urine output, so the registrars in anaesthesia and obstetrics decided that CVP monitoring was indicated. There was difficulty with insertion of the CVP line via the internal jugular route. At the second attempt, neck swelling developed and further attempts were abandoned, particularly as the patient's urine output had improved. Digital pressure was applied to the neck, followed by a pressure dressing. The haematoma extended, and 4 hours later the patient complained of tightness in her neck and inability to breathe. When the anaesthetic registrar arrived the patient was cyanosed and could not breathe at all. Direct laryngoscopy showed an oedematous larynx and pharynx. Several attempts at intubation were made using a bougie, but bradycardia developed and cardiopulmonary resuscitation was required. A senior colleague was called and 100% oxygen was administered, with external cardiac massage and intravenous adrenaline and atropine, but all resuscitation efforts were to no avail.

The CEMD report comments:

> It was reasonable to consider monitoring the CVP. However, the extent of the coagulopathy would be a contraindication to insertion of a neck line, and a long line from the antecubital fossa would have been safer . . . The registrar failed to appreciate the need to watch for airway difficulties after development of the haematoma, and above all to notify the consultant on call . . . It would have been appropriate to transfer her to an ICU (post-operatively).[25]

Vascular damage to carotid, jugular or subclavian vessels may lead to major haemorrhage if manual compression cannot be maintained, especially in the presence of coagulopathy. The conclusion of the CEMD 1991–1993 report in this case was that the use of the central route to establish CVC was contraindicated, but other management options are available.[25] The 1997–1999 report suggested that if a CVC is clinically warranted, coagulation factor transfusion may be given before insertion, and ultrasound-guided CVC insertion is recommended by NICE to reduce the risk of arterial puncture.[5,26] This is discussed in Chapter 5 on haemorrhage. The simpler option of a peripheral-access central venous cannulation ('long line') should not be ignored.

If a woman is having a procedure in the operating theatre, the insertion of a CVC should be strongly considered, as this is an ideal environment in terms of monitoring, layout and assistance.

Pulmonary artery flow-directed catheterisation (PAFC)

The value of PAFC in terms of improving outcomes in critically ill patients remains controversial.[27,28] It might have a place in the management of pre-eclampsia in the ICU to distinguish cardiogenic from non-cardiogenic pulmonary oedema. In past decades there was much debate about the relative merits of using CVP or PCWP to guide cardiovascular management in pre-eclampsia. Cotton *et al.* showed that these two variables correlated, but that PCWP could not be predicted from an individual CVP value.[29,30] However, CVP values within a normal range were rarely associated with excessively high PCWP. Pulmonary oedema has not been reported in pre-eclamptic women with a normal CVP.

Organisation

Organisational problems of management of women who died from pre-eclampsia were not unique to this condition, but were also highlighted in many other causes of death where there was substandard care. The CEMD 1988–1990 report identified delays in management secondary to lack of consultant involvement and/or making clinical decisions. The latter were further subdivided into problems with instituting adequate treatment, delayed delivery in order to achieve fetal maturity (e.g. Case 10) and delayed delivery due to induction of labour rather than delivery by Caesarean section (e.g. Case 2).

Although the consultant referred to in many reports is the obstetrician, the need for involvement of other senior specialists is also often made explicit. In addition to the obstetric anaesthetist, this may include intensive-care specialists, haematologists, renal physicians, obstetric medicine specialists, and general and vascular surgeons. The continuing involvement of the obstetrician in the care of their patient while she is on the ICU is important, as cases of over-hasty discharge from the ICU have occurred.

The NICE Caesarean Section Guideline 2004 suggests that all non-elective Caesarean sections should be performed within 75 minutes of the decision being made.[31] This may be in conflict with the optimum stabilisation of the woman with antihypertensive medication, magnesium and the use of invasive monitoring. Furthermore, the use of steroids to induce fetal lung maturation will take several days. However, delaying delivery must be carefully balanced against maternal safety.

Medical aspects

Chronic hypertension

Chronic hypertension and its associated ischaemic sequelae increasingly compli-cate pregnancy, particularly as maternal age rises. Not infrequently, pre-existing hypertension is associated with pre-eclampsia as term approaches. Renal involvement and obesity are commonly associated with chronic hypertension. Pre-existing hypertension should alert the medical team to the likelihood of complications developing in the third trimester, such that deterioration is identified quickly and treated early. The advantage of this forewarning is offset by the possible development of blood pressure increases that are extremely difficult to control. As has been mentioned earlier, in the section on drug treatment for control of hypertension (*see* page 115), during pregnancy these women are changed from their normal treatment to potentially less effective drugs that do not affect fetal development.

CASE 16 (2000–2002)[4]

A woman with pre-existing hypertension and morbid obesity (BMI > 40 kg/m^2) was booked for shared rather than hospital care. She repeatedly failed to attend for antenatal care, and was not followed up. She was also known to be non-compliant with her antihypertensive medication. At term, she collapsed and died, despite a perimortem Caesarean section performed in the Accident and Emergency department.

This case illustrates a combination of factors resulting in the maternal death of a woman with pre-existing hypertension and obesity. Social issues resulted in a pattern of non-attendance that undoubtedly hampered care. However, the case also highlights failure of communication between midwives and general practitioners.

Phaeochromocytoma

CASE 17 (2000–2002)[4]

A multigravid woman developed hypertension and was admitted near term with headache, blood pressure of 210/100 mmHg, proteinuria (++++) and glycosuria (+++). She was thought to have pre-eclampsia, and labour was induced. Fetal bradycardia led to a 'crash' Caesarean section. The patient was noted to have pulmonary oedema before anaesthesia, and collapsed during surgery. She had several cardiac arrests in the ICU, and died a few hours later.

CASE 18 (1994–1996)[17]

A multigravid woman had an uneventful pregnancy until she was admitted at 37 weeks' gestation with a blood pressure of 170/100 mmHg and headache. She also had proteinuria and was hyper-reflexic, so labour was induced 2 hours later. Two hours after induction, when her blood pressure rose to 210/140 mmHg and she developed visual symptoms, she was delivered by Caesarean section. Liver function tests, uric acid level and platelet count were normal. Because of intense tachycardia and vasoconstriction, phaeochromocytoma was considered at the time of surgery, but nevertheless the patient was returned to the labour ward rather than an ICU for the recovery period. About 2 hours later her blood pressure fell to 70/40 mmHg and she had a terminal cardiac arrest. Autopsy showed that death was due to pulmonary oedema, and that there was an extra-adrenal phaeochromocytoma.

CASE 19 (1994–1996)[17]

This patient complained of headache at 27 weeks' gestation, was found to be hypertensive, and was immediately admitted. Labour was induced for fulminating pre-eclampsia. About 2 hours later there was acute onset of visual disturbance, and her blood pressure was 210/140 mmHg, with fetal tachycardia. An immediate Caesarean section was planned under general anaesthetic. The patient was stable throughout and was extubated at the end of the procedure. She was returned, conscious, to the labour ward, where she became hypotensive 2 hours later, had a cardiac arrest and died.

Phaeochromocytoma is a rare but regular cause of maternal death throughout the series of CEMD reports. It must always be considered in the differential diagnosis of pre-eclampsia, particularly when presentation is atypical. Unfortunately, some antihypertensive drugs may interfere with the diagnostic assays, particularly methyldopa and labetalol.

Blood pressure may be labile and symptoms episodic in the presence of a phaeochromocytoma. If suspected, it must be anticipated that sudden catastrophic cardiopulmonary collapse may occur, particularly at or after delivery. If phaeochromocytoma is diagnosed or suspected, the patient should be managed in a high-dependency unit or ICU until she is stabilised. The involvement of an endocrine surgeon is essential in order to plan the timing of surgical removal in relation to delivery. Attempting to remove a phaeochromocytoma found at the time of Caesarean section or laparotomy in a medically unprepared patient carries an extremely high risk of death.[31, 32]

The following learning points were included in the CEMD 2000–2002 report.[4]

- Phaeochromocytoma should be excluded in multigravid women with severe hypertension with no previous history of pre-eclampsia.
- Glycosuria is a possible pointer towards phaeochromocytoma.
- Phaeochromocytoma can mimic all the features of pre-eclampsia.
- Myocardial damage is a well-recognised complication of phaeochromocytoma.

CHAPTER 7

Cardiac disease

ROBIN RUSSELL

Cardiac disease is one of the leading causes of maternal mortality in the UK. In the most recent CEMD report (2000–2002) it accounted for 44 deaths, the second commonest cause overall.[1] Unlike many direct causes of maternal mortality, for which numbers are fortunately declining, mortality from cardiac disease appears to be on the increase (*see* Figure 7.1). Deaths from cardiac causes may be classified into two groups – congenital and acquired. The leading cause of death in those with congenital heart disease is pulmonary hypertension, while in individuals with acquired heart disease, cardiomyopathy, myocardial infarction and dissection or aneurysm of the thoracic aorta are the commonest causes of death (*see* Table 7.1).[1]

The increase in cardiac deaths is predominantly due to an increase in deaths from acquired heart disease, as those from congenital heart disease have remained fairly constant over the last 40 years. Rheumatic heart disease, historically a common cause

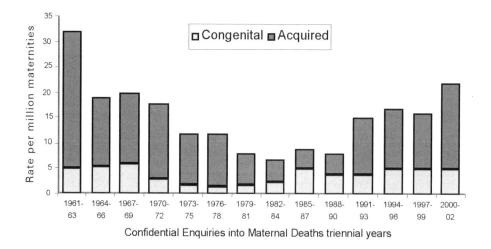

FIGURE 7.1 Maternal mortality from cardiac disease in the UK since 1960.[1]

of acquired death, is now rare and has accounted for only six fatalities in the past 20 years. The increase is related to risk factors such as increasing maternal age, obesity, smoking and hypertension. The increasing number of women with successfully treated congenital heart disease who are now reaching childbearing age also deserves attention. Without appropriate care, further cardiac mortality may result.[2]

TABLE 7.1   Causes of maternal death from cardiac disease in the UK, for the period 1991–2002[1]

CAUSE OF DEATH	TOTAL NUMBER OF DEATHS
Cardiomyopathy/myocarditis	34
Aneurysm of thoracic aorta	28
Myocardial infarction	27
Pulmonary hypertension	22
Others	39
Valvular, including endocarditis	12
Other congenital	9
Sudden adult death syndrome	6
Myocardial fibrosis	4
Other acquired	8
Total	150*

*In five cases the precise cause of death could not be determined.

Pulmonary hypertension

CASE 1 (1997–1999)[3]

A middle-aged woman developed breathlessness in early pregnancy and was found to have primary pulmonary hypertension. She had already lost two of her previous children due to primary pulmonary hypertension, but had not herself been investigated prior to pregnancy. She was appropriately informed that she had a 50% risk of dying in pregnancy, but elected to continue with the pregnancy. She was admitted late in the second trimester in labour, and had a spontaneous vaginal delivery. The child survived, but after being given an intravenous injection of 10 units of oxytocin for the third stage, the patient suffered a cardiac arrest. She was initially resuscitated, but died in the ICU the next day.

| INTERVENTIONS | | PROBLEMS |
OBSTETRIC	ANAESTHETIC	
Multiparous Diagnosed with primary pulmonary hypertension in pregnancy		Deterioration with successive pregnancies Strong family history Not previously investigated
Antenatal counselling		No pre-pregnancy advice Mortality risk of 50%
Admitted in labour at end of second trimester	No antenatal referral or assessment	Lack of multi-disciplinary care No plan for delivery
Spontaneous labour and vaginal delivery		No invasive monitoring
10 units of Syntocinon for management of third stage		Cardiac arrest secondary to fall in systemic vascular resistance

LESSONS

- Such patients should be diagnosed before pregnancy and counselled about the risks of pregnancy.
- Pregnancy, delivery and puerperium should be managed with multidisciplinary input.
- Peripartum management should have included invasive monitoring.
- The significant haemodynamic effects of Syntocinon should have been appreciated and allowed for by administration in a smaller dose over several minutes.

Pulmonary hypertension from whatever cause is associated with a high risk of maternal mortality. The reported death rates are between 30% and 50%. The prognosis is poorer in individuals with a low cardiac index, high right atrial pressure and high pulmonary vascular resistance. The condition may persist after repair of congenital septal defects, or it may be secondary to other conditions, such as thrombo-embolic disease, connective tissue disorders, and certain drugs (e.g. the appetite suppressant fenfluramine). Where no precipitating cause can be found, the condition is known as primary pulmonary hypertension. It is more common in women than in men (ratio of 1.7:1), and usually presents in the third or fourth decade of life.

High mortality is a consequence of the physiological changes of pregnancy and delivery. Increased circulating volume places an added burden on the already compromised right ventricle. This is compounded by pre-existing pulmonary vascular resistance, which is already elevated and fixed, restricting pulmonary flow and increasing right ventricular work. As a consequence, right ventricular failure may be precipitated. Furthermore, reduced systemic vascular resistance may enhance right-to-left shunt in individuals with Eisenmenger's syndrome, worsening gas exchange. Eisenmenger's syndrome, a right-to-left cardiac shunt, develops in those with long-standing left-to-right shunt because of increased pulmonary vascular resistance and pulmonary hypertension secondary to increased pulmonary blood flow. Acidosis and hypercarbia further increase pulmonary vascular resistance, while postpartum haemorrhage leading to hypovolaemia may also result in sudden death. Furthermore, individuals with Eisenmenger's syndrome are at increased risk of endocarditis.

If pulmonary hypertension has not been previously diagnosed, presentation is usually with progressive shortness of breath and fatigue. Effort-associated syncope or haemoptysis can occur, as can chest pain due to right ventricular ischaemia. In pregnancy, deterioration typically occurs in the second trimester as blood volume and cardiac output increase (*see* Figure 7.2). Blood volume increases by 10% during the first trimester of pregnancy, with further rises of 30% and 45% by the end of the second and third trimesters, respectively. This increase is predominantly due to an increase in plasma volume leading to the physiological anaemia of pregnancy.

Auscultation may reveal a pulmonary ejection click and systolic and diastolic murmurs from tricuspid and pulmonary regurgitation. ECG changes are those of right ventricular hypertrophy, namely tall R-waves in the anterior chest leads V1 or V2 with right axis deviation.

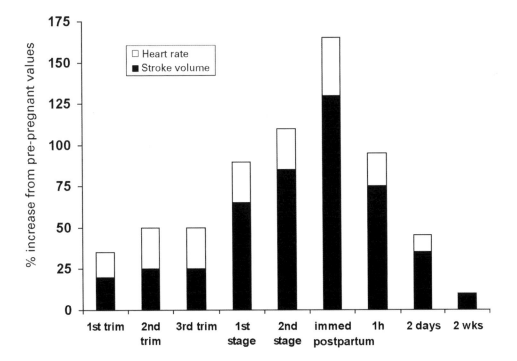

FIGURE 7.2 Changes in cardiac output during pregnancy, labour and puerperium.

The only cure is heart–lung transplantation. Medical treatment aims to reduce pulmonary vascular resistance with oral vasodilators, most commonly calcium-channel blockers or endothelin-receptor antagonists, such as bosentan, although the latter are contraindicated in pregnancy, due to possible teratogenic effects. Supplemental oxygen is beneficial, as pulmonary vascular resistance is reduced. More recent interest has focused on intravenous or nebulised prostacyclin and inhaled nitric oxide. Both agents produce pulmonary vasodilatation, which improves pulmonary pressures in some patients.

In Case 1, the diagnosis of primary pulmonary hypertension was only made once the woman was pregnant, despite the fact that two of her previous children had died from the condition. Primary pulmonary hypertension is known to be familial in some cases, and it is regrettable that this woman had not been previously investigated. If she had been diagnosed and counselled before pregnancy, it is possible that, given a 50% chance of death, she would not have embarked upon this pregnancy. However, once the diagnosis has been made during pregnancy, termination decreases the risk of maternal mortality to less than 10%. Termination was not performed in this case and the pregnancy continued. Unfortunately, the woman presented in spontaneous labour at the end of the second trimester, before she had been seen by all of the relevant specialists, and only during labour was an anaesthetist consulted. The CEMD have repeatedly called for a multi-disciplinary approach to care in high-risk cases through joint management by a consultant obstetrician, cardiologist and anaesthetist so that regular echocardiographic studies are performed. In Case 1 the early onset of labour was predictable, as premature labour is common in these cases and elective hospital admission during the second trimester is recommended.[4]

The principles of management of women with pulmonary hypertension are to avoid the following:[5]
- increases in pulmonary vascular resistance
- decreases in venous return
- decreases in systemic vascular resistance
- myocardial depressants.

There is debate about the most appropriate method of delivery. Availability of appropriately skilled members of staff may be problematic if spontaneous labour is permitted. Vaginal delivery may be preferred, as it avoids the risks of Caesarean section, although this cannot be guaranteed. Induction of labour increases the likelihood that the appropriate staff will be available, but with the added risk that emergency Caesarean section may be required. The use of prostaglandin $F_{2\alpha}$ for induction is best avoided, as it increases pulmonary vascular resistance. Labour should be managed in an environment in which invasive monitoring is available as well as expertise in interpreting haemodynamic parameters and their response to treatment. In most units this is the intensive-care unit. Direct arterial monitoring allows continuous blood pressure reading and a means of regularly assessing the acid–base balance, while a CVP line permits measurement of right atrial pressure. There is controversy regarding the place of pulmonary artery catheters in the management of labour, as their use does not appear to improve outcome.[6] Pulmonary artery pressure and vascular resistance can be measured, but catheter insertion is not without risks, especially of thrombosis and pulmonary artery rupture.

For those who labour, early epidural analgesia using low-dose local anaesthetic and opioid solution is now considered beneficial.[7] However, its use is reported mainly in patients with Eisenmenger's syndrome, in whom changes in pulmonary vascular resistance are better tolerated, as the defect allows pressure increases to be transmitted to the left side of the heart. Well-conducted regional analgesia blunts the physiological response to painful contractions without having a significant effect on systemic vascular resistance. Moreover, elective instrumental delivery, to prevent a prolonged second stage, is facilitated. Third-stage management is crucial, as is demonstrated by the current case. Syntocinon injection has profound haemodynamic effects caused by relaxation of vascular smooth muscle. A sudden decrease in systemic vascular resistance may produce severe maternal hypotension. Cardiac arrest may result, and successful resuscitation may not be possible. The dose of 10 units of Syntocinon is twice that now recommended by the *British National Formulary*, which also states that in severe cardiovascular disease the drug is contraindicated. If Syntocinon is to be used, it must be infused slowly with the haemodynamic response closely observed. A 5-unit intravenous bolus over 5–10 minutes may be followed by an infusion of 40 units over 4 hours. In severe cases Syntocinon may be omitted, although the risk of postpartum haemorrhage is increased.

Elective Caesarean section allows the timing of delivery to be predicted. The decision as to whether to use general or regional anaesthesia is another source of debate. For example, regional anaesthesia may significantly reduce systemic vascular resistance, and therefore may be considered unsuitable. However, successful use of both epidural and combined spinal–epidural anaesthesia has been reported.[8,9] General anaesthesia is also not without risk. Laryngoscopy and intubation may further elevate pulmonary artery pressure, although this can be attenuated with the use of an opioid-based technique. Positive pressure ventilation may have a detrimental effect on venous return and may further elevate pulmonary vascular resistance, as may lung hyperinflation. Cardiac failure is a potential consequence. Nitrous oxide is probably best avoided, as it can also increase pulmonary vascular resistance. A possible advantage of general anaesthesia is that tracheal intubation facilitates the use of inhaled nitric oxide. As with labour, and regardless of the anaesthetic technique, invasive monitoring is required throughout. Effective postoperative pain relief is necessary to prevent excessive release of maternal catecholamines which may further increase pulmonary vascular resistance.

Venous thromboembolism is a significant risk for individuals with pulmonary hypertension, and postnatal anticoagulation is widely recommended, especially following Caesarean section under general anaesthesia (*see* Chapter 8A). However, cyanotic patients not infrequently have intrinsic bleeding problems, so treatment should be considered carefully.

Aortic aneurysm dissection

CASE 2 (2000–2002)[1]

An obese woman, who had been well during pregnancy, developed crushing chest pain radiating to her back near term. She was started on low-molecular-weight heparin in case she had suffered a pulmonary embolism, but this was discontinued when standard investigations were found to be normal. No diagnosis was made, and she was sent home some days later. When reviewed in the antenatal clinic she seemed better, but she died shortly afterwards from a ruptured aortic aneurysm, which had dissected into the pericardium.

INTERVENTIONS		PROBLEMS
OBSTETRIC	ANAESTHETIC	
Obesity		Inadequate investigation
Crushing chest pain radiating to back		Diagnosed as pulmonary embolism
		Treated with anticoagulants
Investigations did not confirm diagnosis of pulmonary embolism		No further investigation of central chest pain
		Failure to consult other disciplines
Review in antenatal clinic		Problem ignored as symptoms improved
Sudden death		Ruptured aortic aneurysm

LESSONS

- The diagnosis of aortic dissection should be considered when no other cause for chest pain has been found.
- Central chest pain in pregnancy should be investigated sufficiently to identify its cause.
- Family members should be screened for associated diseases (e.g. Marfan's syndrome, Ehlers–Danlos syndrome).

Although it is considered to be a rare cause of maternal mortality, in the last 10 years in the UK dissecting aortic aneurysm has accounted for a similar number of deaths to pulmonary hypertension, myocardial infarction and cardiomyopathy. Indeed, as many as 50% of those women under 40 years old who develop the condition do so in pregnancy. Predisposing factors include Marfan's and Ehlers–Danlos syndromes, coarctation of the aorta and bicuspid aortic valves. In up to 50% of cases hypertension is present. Histology reveals medial degeneration of the aortic wall with intimal tears occurring in the regions subjected to greatest pressure fluctuations. In pregnancy, acute dissection is most common in the ascending aorta.

For women who are known to be at increased risk of dissection because of predisposing factors, pre-pregnancy assessment is recommended. If there is no evidence of cardiac failure and the aortic root diameter is less than 4 cm (normal value 2.2 cm), pregnancy is usually tolerated well. If the aortic root diameter is greater than 4 cm, the patient should be counselled about the risks of dissection. During pregnancy, regular echocardiography, with measurement of aortic root size, and strict control of hypertension are necessary.

The clinical manifestations of acute aortic dissection are well documented and reflect the site of the tear.[10] Nearly all of them present with sudden-onset severe back or chest pain that is classically described as stabbing or tearing. Aortic valve involvement that produces regurgitation may occur in up to 50% of cases, and coronary artery flow may be compromised. Obstruction of branches of the aorta can produce organ ischaemia. The diagnosis of acute aortic dissection is frequently missed at first presentation, as in this case and many others reported to the CEMD. However, delay in diagnosis is not always associated with poor outcome.[11] Thorough investigation is required to exclude other possible causes of severe chest pain, such as pulmonary embolism and myocardial infarction. Chest X-ray shows a widened mediastinum in 50% of cases. Concerns about exposure to radiation are overstated when dealing with potentially life-threatening situations. ECG changes are non-specific, most commonly involving ST segments and T-waves. Transthoracic echocardiography is more useful, but may still miss 20% of cases due to technical limitations. These are overcome using trans-oesophageal echocardiography, although an experienced operator is required. Alternatively, CT or MRI scanning may aid diagnosis.[12]

In Case 2, few details are provided about the investigations that were performed. It is unlikely that these included echocardiography, and it appears that once the diagnosis of pulmonary embolism had been excluded and the patient's symptoms improved, further tests that might have helped to diagnose an aortic dissection were not carried out. Once again it should be emphasised that if women present with either symptoms or signs suggestive of cardiac disease, a full cardiovascular assessment should be made.

Surgical intervention is required for dissection of ascending aorta, and without treatment over 50% of cases die within 48 hours. However, it is of interest that a number of women who were reported to the CEMD presented several days or weeks before their demise. It is therefore vital that staff consider the diagnosis of aortic dissection in women who present with chest pain, especially if there is associated hypertension.[13] Surgery is not without considerable risk, but may lead to a successful outcome. Before 28 weeks' gestation it has been recommended that aortic repair should proceed with the fetus *in utero*. After 32 weeks, Caesarean section is performed immediately before aortic repair.[14] Between 28 and 32 weeks the decision with regard to timing of delivery should be based on the health of the fetus.

It has been recommended that post-mortem histological examination of the aorta should be performed. Medial degeneration, although normal in pregnancy, may signify Marfan's syndrome, which needs to be excluded. Other family members should be screened.

Cardiomyopathy

CASE 3 (1997–1999)[3]

A morbidly obese woman was admitted to hospital at the end of her pregnancy, complaining of breathlessness. Pulmonary embolus and deep vein thrombosis were apparently excluded. The patient developed hypertension, proteinuria and tachycardia of 120 beats/min. All of these features were thought to be due to pre-eclampsia. Delivery by Caesarean section was planned because of transverse lie. The anaesthetist had considered echocardiography, but decided against the request because the patient was so obese. Invasive monitoring during the planned delivery had to be abandoned because of difficulty in siting the lines. During the induction of anaesthesia the patient suffered a cardiac arrest and died. Autopsy showed that she had a dilated enlarged heart, thought to be due to puerperal cardiomyopathy. She also had a kidney tumour that may have been the cause of the hypertension and proteinuria, although pre-eclampsia is a more likely cause.

INTERVENTIONS		PROBLEMS
OBSTETRIC	ANAESTHETIC	
Obesity Breathlessness at end of pregnancy		Deep vein thrombosis and pulmonary embolism excluded No further investigation
Hypertension, proteinuria and tachycardia		Diagnosis of pre-eclampsia No further investigation of symptoms
Planned Caesarean section for transverse lie	First seen by anaesthetist on day of surgery	Lack of multi-disciplinary care
	Echocardiography not performed	Inadequate pre-operative investigation
	Attempts at invasive monitoring abandoned	Failure to seek help from more experienced staff
	Induction of general anaesthesia	Cardiac arrest and death

LESSONS

- A diagnosis of cardiomyopathy should be considered in individuals with significant breathlessness and tachycardia.
- Full cardiovascular assessment, including echocardiography, is needed for those with symptoms and signs suggestive of cardiac pathology.
- Multi-disciplinary care is needed.
- Adequate advance notice of high-risk cases should be given to obstetric anaesthetists.
- Invasive monitoring should be sited before induction of anaesthesia in high-risk cases.
- Assistance should be sought from anaesthetic colleagues when dealing with problem cases.

Cardiomyopathy may be divided into dilated and restrictive types. The majority of pregnancy-related deaths result from dilated cardiomyopathy. With regard to the deaths reported to the CEMD, puerperal cardiomyopathy is the commonest cause. This dilated cardiomyopathy of uncertain aetiology presents in either the last month of pregnancy or within 6 months of delivery in women not previously known to have heart disease. The precise aetiology has not yet been established, although an immunological basis seems likely. The condition is more common in multiple pregnancy, and there is often associated hypertension. The incidence of puerperal cardiomyopathy in the UK is less than 1 in 5,000.[15]

The presentation of puerperal cardiomyopathy depends on the degree of ventricular dysfunction. Dyspnoea and tachycardia may be early signs, as in Case 3. However, these signs are somewhat non-specific, and further investigation is required in order to make the diagnosis. In more severe cases hypotension may develop and there may be evidence of left ventricular failure. Examination may reveal a third heart sound, a gallop rhythm or basal crackles. ECG features are variable, and include sinus tachycardia, ectopic beats or arrhythmias. In severe cases, pulmonary oedema is seen on chest X-ray. Echocardiography is helpful and may demonstrate dilation involving all four chambers, but in particular left ventricular dysfunction. Mortality is usually due to pulmonary or cerebral embolism, although it may occasionally follow the injudicious use of general anaesthesia, as in Case 3.

A number of key recommendations highlighted in the CEMD report were not followed in this case. No information is provided about multi-disciplinary care of this high-risk pregnancy, which suggests that it did not occur. It appears that a diagnosis of pre-eclampsia was made and no further investigations were performed and no clinicians from other specialties were involved. Given the features of obesity, breathlessness, hypertension, proteinuria and tachycardia, this is disappointing.

Although a non-urgent Caesarean section for transverse lie was planned, it was not until the day of surgery that the patient was first assessed by an anaesthetist. Whether this represents a failure on the part of the obstetricians in not informing the obstetric anaesthetic service is not certain. In high-risk cases, sufficient notice must be given to ensure that there is adequate time for consultation, investigation and assembly of appropriate resources.[1,3] Having seen the woman on the day of surgery, the anaesthetist did not insist that echocardiography was performed because of anticipated technical difficulties due to maternal obesity. This is again disappointing, given the patient's history, as echocardiography can provide useful information that may influence anaesthetic technique. Had the results of echocardiography been available in this case, greater efforts might have been made to place arterial and central venous catheters before inducing anaesthesia. The CEMD have stressed the importance of invasive monitoring in individuals with cardiovascular disease.[1,3] Furthermore, it has been recommended that when specialist skills are required, such as placing lines in challenging patients, anaesthetists should not hesitate to call upon the assistance of other colleagues. As cardiac arrest followed induction of general anaesthesia, it appears likely that this woman had significant cardiovascular compromise from her cardiomyopathy, and we can only speculate as to whether more thorough pre-operative work-up would have resulted in a better outcome.

It is also noteworthy that no histology was performed at the autopsy. Again this does not follow the guidance in the CEMD report, which states that histology should be undertaken in all cases of maternal death unless there are positive reasons for not following such action. Indeed, in this case the pathology assessor's report cast some doubt on the validity of the diagnosis of cardiomyopathy.

Ischaemic heart disease

CASE 4 (1997–1999)[3]

A woman who rarely attended for antenatal care was known to have had hypertension in each of her previous pregnancies, and to have a family history of ischaemic heart disease. During her last pregnancy she had sustained systolic hypertension (170–180 mmHg) but no action was taken, perhaps because her diastolic blood pressure was about 75 mmHg. Just before term she collapsed and died. The autopsy showed severe coronary atheroma without actual infarction, and 'massive' left ventricular hypertrophy, presumably due to long-standing hypertension.

INTERVENTIONS		PROBLEMS
OBSTETRIC	ANAESTHETIC	
Poor attendance for antenatal care		Risk factor for maternal morbidity/mortality
Known hypertension + family history of ischaemic heart disease		Increased risk of maternal and neonatal morbidity/mortality
Previous untreated blood pressure of 170–180/75 mmHg		Lack of awareness of importance of high systolic and mean blood pressure

---

LESSONS

- A diagnosis of ischaemic heart disease should be considered if risk factors are present.
- Recommendations for providing antenatal care for poor attenders should be followed to improve compliance.
- All healthcare workers, but particularly midwives, need to be aware of the importance of both systolic and diastolic blood pressure.
- Resuscitation skills are mandatory for those providing obstetric care.

Ischaemic heart disease and myocardial infarction are uncommon in the pregnant population, and there have been few published cases. However, this situation seems likely to change, as the risk factors are increasing. Risk factors include the following:

- older age at which women choose to have children
- smoking
- diabetes
- obesity
- cocaine abuse.

Most infarcts occur in the third trimester, peripartum or postpartum. Not all are associated with atheromatous coronary artery disease with both dissection and spasm implicated. Mortality from infarction is of the order of 19%.[16]

Women with known myocardial ischaemia or infarction require multi-disciplinary care. Physiological changes of pregnancy and labour put an additional stress on the already compromised myocardium, and may precipitate further ischaemia. Associated problems such as hypertension and anaemia should be addressed. Elective Caesarean section does not appear to improve outcome, and operative delivery is indicated only for obstetric reasons. In labour, regional analgesia is recommended in order to minimise sympathetic outflow and facilitate elective instrumental delivery.

The above case of unexpected collapse and death in a woman with severe coronary artery disease and hypertension raises a number of issues. Although the risk factors for ischaemic heart disease were known, antenatal care as recommended by the CEMD did not appear to occur. At the booking visit, a risk and needs assessment should take place to ensure that every woman is offered suitable antenatal care. Given this patient's history of long-standing hypertension, consultant care with regular clinic visits was appropriate. Her poor clinic attendance further increased her risk. The CEMD found that in 20% of maternal mortalities the patient booked late or missed over four routine antenatal visits. Given these risk factors, every effort should have been made to ensure clinic attendance and to provide information on the risk of hypertension in pregnancy. Whether this patient's attendance at clinic would have improved if she had been told of the risk to her own health and that of the baby is a matter for speculation.

Diastolic blood pressure has in the past been used as a gauge of the severity of pre-eclampsia. However, excessive systolic blood pressure is thought to be a cause of intracerebral bleeding, so current guidelines now identify systolic pressure above which treatment is indicated. This does not appear to have occurred in the above case. Finally, this unfortunate case is a timely reminder of the need for all staff who provide antenatal care to keep their resuscitation skills up to date.

Medical management

Physiological changes within the cardiovascular system during pregnancy are significant, and may lead to functional deterioration in certain conditions. Cardiac output increases by 40% by the end of the second trimester, through increases in both stroke volume and heart rate. In response to a reduction in afterload, resulting from systemic vasodilatation, blood volume also increases during pregnancy by up to 40%. Central venous and pulmonary capillary wedge pressures remain unchanged, although the reduction in serum colloid osmotic pressure increases the likelihood of pulmonary oedema.

Labour further increases cardiac output. This is in response to both pain and expulsion of blood from the intervillous space during uterine contractions. The former may be minimised with effective analgesia. The large autotransfusion at delivery results in an even greater stress on the cardiovascular system, with cardiac output increasing to levels in excess of 150% of those seen prior to pregnancy.

The above vignettes from the CEMD represent cases with poor outcome. Efforts to decrease maternal mortality focus on pre-pregnancy counselling, antenatal multi-disciplinary care, management of labour and delivery, and postnatal follow-up. However, not all women with cardiac disease may be recognised, since some may only have their condition discovered at autopsy.

Pre-pregnancy counselling

This allows a formal risk assessment and optimisation of cardiovascular pathology.[17] However, some women minimise their symptoms in an effort to seek medical approval. Others may rely on interpreters who may not pass on the relevant details, especially where there is conflict with a desire for the woman to have a child. Conditions such as pulmonary hypertension, severe left ventricular failure, left-sided obstruction and dilated aortic root all have a poor prognosis, and pregnancy is not advisable.[18] Pre-pregnancy counselling also allows fetal outcome to be discussed. For individuals with congenital heart disease there is a risk that the baby will inherit a similar condition, and for those with maternal cyanotic conditions, fetal development may be compromised.

Pre-pregnancy counselling also provides the opportunity to review maternal drug therapy. Although most drugs are relatively safe, some (e.g. angiotensin-converting-enzyme inhibitors, warfarin, amiodarone, spironolactone) may need to be changed.[2]

Multi-disciplinary antenatal care

The skills of experienced obstetricians, cardiologists, midwives and anaesthetists in regional centres are vital to achieving a good outcome. In some situations it may be prudent to discuss termination of pregnancy if continuation represents a greater risk to the mother.

Anaesthesia for termination of pregnancy also carries a significant risk. Although the physiological changes seen in the cardiovascular system in pregnancy are not as pronounced in early pregnancy, the problems associated with the underlying disease require careful evaluation. A thorough pre-operative assessment, with appropriate multi-disciplinary input, should provide a guide as to whether general or regional anaesthesia is more suitable. Given the nature of the procedure, general anaesthesia is more often used. Invasive monitoring, placed before induction of anaesthesia, should be employed where necessary. During the first trimester intubation may not be required, thereby simplifying the anaesthetic technique. Carefully titrated total intravenous anaesthesia avoids the need for volatile agents, with their tocolytic effects, and nitrous oxide, which may increase pulmonary vascular resistance. Syntocinon may not be required for termination in early pregnancy, and is probably best withheld. Depending on the severity of the underlying condition, postoperative care on a high-dependency or intensive-care unit may be indicated.

Diagnosis of cardiac disease in pregnancy may be difficult, as a number of the symptoms and signs may be present in normal pregnancy.[19] Fatigue, breathlessness, tachycardia and oedema need not necessarily signify cardiac failure. However, chest pain, arrhythmias, hypotension and pulmonary oedema all warrant further investigation. Regular assessment throughout each trimester of pregnancy, looking for any deterioration in condition, is necessary.[7] Further investigation or referral may be required, as may hospital admission.

Case conferences

For case conferences, the most important issue to be agreed is whether it is preferable for the baby to be born by vaginal delivery or elective Caesarean section. Unfortunately, it is always possible that emergency Caesarean section may be necessary if vaginal delivery is planned. If immediate operative delivery is required, the anaesthetic risk may be considerable and, in order to avoid this difficult situation, elective surgery may be chosen even though this may be of greater risk than vaginal delivery. Faced with such a dilemma, the likelihood of successful spontaneous birth should be balanced against the increased risks of surgery. The risk of intervention is increased if labour is induced, and where possible this should be avoided. However, spontaneous labour is unpredictable, and relevant clinicians may not always be available. The location of delivery should be decided. For labour, the choice lies between the delivery suite and a high-dependency or intensive-care unit. The latter may be preferred if invasive monitoring is to be used, although midwifery and obstetric staff need to be in attendance. If elective Caesarean section is planned, this may be performed on the delivery suite. However, if the high-dependency or intensive-care unit is not in close proximity, the location of surgery may need to be reviewed.

Aortocaval compression should be avoided at all times, especially when regional analgesia or anaesthesia is used. Antibiotic prophylaxis to minimise the risk of endocarditis should be considered, and the possibility of thromboembolic complications should be assessed and suitable prophylaxis planned.

Anticoagulation

For labour and vaginal delivery, provided that the mother is not fully anticoagulated, low-dose epidural analgesia is recommended for nearly all cases.[7] If heparin has been given during pregnancy, its use in the peripartum period should be planned in advance, balancing the risk of thromboembolic complications against those of postpartum haemorrhage and excessive bleeding during operative delivery. Recognised guidelines on the use of heparin and regional blocks should be followed.[20] If regional analgesia is used in labour, a continuous infusion may be preferable to intermittent top-ups, as fluctuations in blood pressure are minimised. However, block height should be checked regularly to prevent an inappropriately high sympathetic block, which may itself cause hypotension.

Monitoring

Invasive haemodynamic monitoring is frequently used. Direct arterial blood pressure measurement provides a continuous record that may be valuable when vasoactive drugs are used, or if significant haemorrhage is anticipated. CVP monitoring may be helpful for assessing preload, especially in individuals who are sensitive to hypovolaemia. However, caution should be exercised with regard to over-reliance on values in the presence of pre-eclampsia, as low colloid osmotic pressure and endothelial damage to pulmonary vessels may result in pulmonary oedema following even minimal fluid challenges.

Delivery and management of the third stage

Management of the third stage of labour poses further dilemmas. Intravenous boluses of Syntocinon may cause profound cardiovascular instability[21] due to their ability to cause a significant reduction in systemic vascular resistance, and they have been associated with maternal mortality. Reduced doses are now recommended, but even these, in the presence of significant cardiac disease, may cause profound haemodynamic instability. Withholding Syntocinon increases the risk of haemorrhage due to uterine atony, which may be equally dangerous. A slow bolus and infusion, such as 5 units in 5–10 minutes followed by 40 units in 500 ml over 4–5 hours, has been recommended, although in severe disease even this is best omitted.[7] In some patients, ergometrine may be a suitable alternative, although it causes vasoconstriction, rendering it unsuitable for use in pulmonary or systemic hypertension and ischaemic heart disease.

Delivery is often a time when the focus of attention switches from mother to baby. This is unwise, as dramatic changes in maternal cardiovascular physiology take place, most notably the significant autotransfusion from uterine contraction. For a woman with limited cardiac reserve this may be sufficient to precipitate left ventricular failure and pulmonary oedema. Fluid balance is crucial in the immediate postpartum period, to ensure adequate filling pressures while avoiding overload. Adequate pain relief following delivery, especially if there has been significant perineal trauma, reduces sympathetic outflow, which may have a detrimental effect on cardiovascular function. Paracetamol, with or without codeine phosphate, and non-steroidal anti-inflammatory drugs may be given either orally or rectally if there are no contraindications. Continued monitoring of pulse, blood pressure, respiratory rate and oxygen saturation should be continued after delivery. Supplemental oxygen may be necessary to maintain adequate saturation. An assessment of the risk of thromboembolism should be made, and where necessary heparin should be given.[22]

Regional analgesia

Elective instrumental delivery performed under effective regional analgesia minimises the cardiovascular instability that may complicate prolonged pushing. The Valsalva manoeuvre reduces venous return, which activates the baroreceptor reflex, causing tachycardia and vasoconstriction. An uncomplicated lift-out delivery can usually be performed with analgesia provided by a low-dose local anaesthetic with opioid epidural top-up. More concentrated local anaesthetic solutions, such as those used for Caesarean section, are more likely to produce maternal hypotension.

Caesarean section

Both regional and general anaesthesia have been used in most cardiac conditions. It is possibly the care with which either is administered, rather than the technique itself, that dictates outcome.[7] A number of issues may influence which technique is preferred (see Table 7.2). Invasive monitoring is usually advised, and this should be sited before induction. If regional anaesthesia is chosen, an incremental technique using an epidural, sequential combined spinal–epidural or spinal catheter provides greater haemodynamic stability than a single-shot spinal injection. As with vaginal delivery, management of the third stage carries the risk of both cardiovascular collapse and excessive haemorrhage, and consequently oxytocic drugs must be used with great caution. Postoperative care on a high-dependency or intensive-care unit is recommended.

TABLE 7.2   Choice of anaesthetic technique for Caesarean section in the cardiac patient[7]

FACTORS THAT FAVOUR REGIONAL ANAESTHETIC	FACTORS THAT FAVOUR GENERAL ANAESTHETIC
Negative inotropic effect of general anaesthesia	Significant reduction in SVR with surgical anaesthesia
Stress response to laryngoscopy producing acute pulmonary hypertension	Risk of arrhythmias requiring DC cardioversion
Possibility of maternal death	Anxiety-related cyanosis or pulmonary hypertension
Chance to see baby	Need for postoperative ventilation or further intervention, such as cardiac surgery
Anticipated difficult airway	
	Impaired coagulation or recent administration of anticoagulants

General anaesthesia has traditionally been used for Caesarean section in cardiac patients, as it has been considered to provide greater haemodynamic stability, although intra-operative blood loss is greater. However, laryngoscopy and intubation can result in a dramatic increase in maternal catecholamine release. If general anaesthesia is used, laryngeal reflexes should be obtunded. A number of techniques for minimising the stress response to laryngoscopy have been described, and of these the use of an opioid-based induction is probably the most appropriate. Recently, the use of remifentanil has been demonstrated to be effective.[23]

Bacterial endocarditis

Antibiotic prophylaxis against bacterial endocarditis should be considered for women who may be susceptible. Amoxicillin and gentamicin are usually given to individuals with prosthetic heart valves or a history of endocarditis. For other cardiac conditions, the risk of endocarditis should be assessed and antibiotics used at the discretion of those responsible for management of labour. Clindamycin may be used for individuals who are sensitive to penicillin.

Other issues

Evidence-based recommendations on best management of complex cardiac cases are difficult to find, and care is usually largely based on small series or personal opinions. Thus in 1996 the UK Obstetric Anaesthetists' Association set up a central registry for reporting the outcome of high-risk pregnancy.[24] Such national data collection may aid decision making when faced with rare complex cardiac disease.

Finally, given the relative rarity of cardiac arrest in maternity units, the CEMD have recommended that all medical and midwifery staff should be trained in resuscitation to an appropriate level. Regular drills for maternal resuscitation should be performed, and attendance at specialised courses such as *Managing Obstetric Emergencies and Trauma (MOET)*[25] and *Advanced Life Support in Obstetrics (ALSO)*[26] should be encouraged.

Thromboembolism

GORDON LYONS AND MITKO KOCAREV

Deep venous thrombosis (DVT) and pulmonary embolism (PE) are leading causes of maternal mortality during pregnancy and the puerperium in the developed world. Pregnancy is a physiologically prothrombotic state and therefore a major contributing factor. Early recognition, diagnosis and treatment of thromboembolism reduce morbidity and mortality. Many of these deaths are sudden and occur outside hospital. Anaesthetists may become involved in the critical care of an acute event, and in turn anticoagulation management may influence the choice of anaesthetic technique. Even when pregnancy and delivery are uneventful, the anaesthetist may take responsibility for ensuring postpartum thromboprophylaxis.

Thrombi may form in any of the following:

- ileo-femoral veins
- veins of the calf
- superficial veins and venous system of the upper limbs
- cerebral veins
- pelvic sepsis (thrombophlebitis) – this is infrequent, but triggers thrombosis in the ovarian vein with extension into the inferior vena cava and renal vein.

Incidence and risk factors

The true incidence is uncertain, due to under-reporting and failure to provide objective testing. From 1952, the CEMD have provided comprehensive data on mortality from thromboembolic events.[1] During the early decades, mortality decreased, particularly after vaginal delivery, while the absolute number of deaths following Caesarean section and during the antenatal and intrapartum period has not changed significantly. However, when recent increases in the Caesarean section rate are taken into account, the implication is that deaths from thromboembolism have declined. The last published report, covering the triennium 2000–2002, listed 26 deaths from pulmonary embolism, which represents an incidence of 1.3 in 100,000 maternities.[1]

Pregnancy is prothrombotic to the extent that the risk of DVT is elevated up to 10-fold compared with that for non-pregnant women of comparable age.[2] PE develops in approximately 24% of pregnant women with untreated DVT, with a subsequent mortality rate of 15%.[3] Some reports suggest that antenatal DVT is more common than postnatal DVT,[4] but the accuracy of these findings is uncertain, as some women presenting with postnatal DVT might not be referred to the obstetric services.[5] One retrospective study showed that the calculated risk of venous thromboembolism was about 3 to 8 times higher postpartum then antepartum.[6] A meta-analysis of 14 relevant studies on DVT in pregnancy or the puerperium suggests that the estimated relative distribution of 100 DVT events was 0.23 per day during pregnancy and 0.82 per day in the postpartum period, with a 15-fold higher risk during the puerperium.[7]

Advanced maternal age and operative delivery are major risk factors for the development of DVT.[5] The incidence of clinically diagnosed DVT is estimated to be 0.08–1.2% following vaginal delivery, increasing to 2.2–3.0% after Caesarean section.[4] It has been suggested that women with previous episodes of venous thromboembolism are at increased risk, with a recurrence rate of 10–14% during the subsequent pregnancy.[8] Other common risk factors for venous thromboembolism in pregnancy include weight over 80 kg, prolonged immobilisation, gross varicose veins, dehydration, pre-eclampsia, multiple gestation, infective and inflammatory conditions (e.g. inflammatory bowel disease, urinary tract infections), major obstetric haemorrhage, and certain medical conditions (e.g. nephrotic syndrome, thrombophilia).[9]

CASE 1 (1997–1999)[10]

An overweight woman aged over 30 years and with a strong family history of thromboembolic disease developed thrombophlebitis and was admitted to the Accident and Emergency department at eight weeks' gestation with chest pain. The GP had suggested a diagnosis of PE, but a medical registrar believed that chest X-ray and anticoagulation were contraindicated by pregnancy, and the woman was allowed home with a diagnosis of musculoskeletal pain. Three days later she saw the GP, who thought that PE had been excluded. Two days later, the patient attended hospital with classic symptoms, including haemoptysis. She was transferred to a major centre where the clinical picture was considered 'not typical' of PE. A V/Q scan was arranged for the following day, but the patient died before this was done.

This case illustrates some of the risk factors for PE, which were unfortunately ignored. The GP's clinical diagnosis was overridden for erroneous reasons. Added to this there were communication failures, and the recommended chest X-ray did not present a great risk to the fetus.

Deep vein thrombosis

Physiology

Virchow's triad is still considered to be the primary mechanism involved in the development of this disease. It consists of the following:

- hypercoagulability
- venous stasis
- vascular damage.

A physiological increase in coagulation activity relative to fibrinolytic activity during pregnancy reflects preparation for the haemostatic challenge of delivery. This includes an increase in the activity of several procoagulant factors, namely I, II, V, VII, VIII, X and von Willebrand factor.[5] At the same time, resistance to the endogenous anticoagulant-activated protein C develops, and levels of protein S, which is a cofactor for protein C, decrease. The fibrinolytic system is also inhibited by increased concentrations of plasminogen activator inhibitor 1 and particularly inhibitor 2, which is derived from the placenta.[5]

Increased venous stasis, which is apparent by the end of the first trimester and most obvious at 36 weeks,[11] is the most constant predisposing factor. Venous distensibility and capacitance increase as a result of pregnancy-related hormonal changes. Compression of the inferior vena cava by the gravid uterus, and particularly compression of the left common iliac vein by the left common iliac artery, which crosses the vein only on the left side, worsen the situation. This may account for the predominance of deep venous thrombosis in the left leg. Several reports suggest that in almost 90% of pregnant women the left side was affected, compared with 55% of non-pregnant women.[5,7]

Vascular injury during vaginal delivery, but especially during surgical delivery, causes endothelial damage, and activates coagulation activity with subsequent development of vascular thrombosis.

CASE 2 (1997–1999)[10]

An obese primigravida had a breech presentation diagnosed at 34 weeks. At just over 36 weeks she was admitted with ruptured membranes, and underwent Caesarean section. She went home on day 4 with a haemoglobin level of 8.4 g%. The next day the midwife noted that she was breathless and had pain in her upper back. The GP visited her at home. On day 6 she collapsed at home, and despite intensive-care treatment she died 2 weeks later.

As with other causes of death described in this book, obesity is a significant issue. In Case 2, obesity and delivery by Caesarean section were risk factors for PE. There is no mention of the thromboprophylaxis regimen used.

Thrombophilias

The physiological coagulation system represents a balance between procoagulants and anticoagulants. Any change in this balance in favour of coagulation has the potential to promote deep vein thrombosis.

Thrombophilias are a group of heritable or acquired disorders that predispose to thrombosis. Up to 15% of the population may suffer from thrombophilia,[12] and the latter is implicated in approximately 50% of all thrombotic events in pregnancy and the puerperium.[13] The prevalence rates for thrombophilia in a European population are listed in Table 8A.1.[14]

TABLE 8A.1 Typical prevalence rates for thrombophilia in a European population.[14] Reprinted with permission from Elsevier.

THROMBOPHILIC DEFECT	PREVALENCE (PER 1,000 POPULATION)
MTHFR C-677→T homozygosity	100
Factor V Leiden	20–70
Lupus inhibitors	30
Anticardiolipin antibodies	30
Prothrombin 20210A	20
Antithrombin deficiency	2.5–5.5
Protein C deficiency	2.0–3.3

MTHFR, methylene tetrahydrofolate reductase.

Inherited thrombophilias

Genetic influence is important, and may not be apparent until pregnancy. Deficiencies of the physiological anticoagulants antithrombin III, protein C and protein S are inherited in an autosomal-dominant pattern. Antithrombin III deficiency is the most thrombogenic, but is uncommon, and the associated risk of thromboembolism in pregnant women who are not receiving anticoagulant treatment is about 30%.[15] Asymptomatic women with protein C or protein S deficiency have an eightfold increased risk of pregnancy-related thromboembolism, but most thromboembolic events occur postpartum.[16]

Resistance to activated protein C caused by an adenine-506-guanine mutation in factor V (referred to as factor V Leiden) is found in around 20–30% of women with pregnancy-associated thromboembolism, and in up to 50% of those with recurrent thromboembolic events.[13]

A common variation in a prothrombin gene, described as a guanine-20210-adenine mutation, has been associated with elevated plasma prothrombin levels and an increased risk of development of thromboembolism and cerebral vein thrombosis.[13]

Hyperhomocysteinemia linked with homozygosity for the cytosine-677-thymine mutation in the gene encoding 5,10-methylenetetrahydrofolate reductase (MTHFR), which plays an important role in the metabolism of homocysteine, is recognised as another risk factor for venous thrombosis.[17] Reduced MTHFR activity together with elevated plasma homocysteine levels can be found in 5–15% of the population.[13] Homocysteine, which promotes vascular damage, is an independent risk factor for all types of vascular disease. However, a recent systematic review failed to demonstrate an increased risk of venous thromboembolism in pregnant women who were homozygous for MTHFR, compared with non-pregnant women.[18] The mechanism is uncertain, but one explanation is linked to the administration of folic acid supplements in pregnancy, which might reduce the level of homocysteine.[18]

Not all pregnant women with hereditary thrombophilias will develop venous thromboembolism.[19] This strongly suggests that thrombosis in this group of patients is a multi-causal event, involving both genetic and acquired risk factors. In women with multiple or homozygous thrombophilic defects, the risk is increased two- to threefold.[20]

Acquired thrombophilia

Antiphospholipid syndrome is an acquired autoimmune disorder characterised by a persistently increased level of specific circulating lupus anticoagulant or anticardiolipin antibodies, and associated recurrent venous or arterial thrombosis. The risk of recurrent thromboses in affected women is increased by 70%,[21] and is possibly higher than this during pregnancy, but strong evidence is not currently available.

Clinical manifestations

Clinical findings of pain or discomfort, tenderness and leg swelling were reported in 85% of pregnant women with DVT.[22] Pelvic thrombosis should be included in the differential diagnosis if low abdominal pain, increased temperature and increased white cell count are presenting features.

Leg pain and swelling are common manifestations during pregnancy. In addition, some affected patients might be clinically asymptomatic. Because unrecognised and untreated DVT is a potentially lethal event, vigilance should be maintained.

Diagnosis

The clinical diagnosis of DVT in pregnancy is not reliable. When consecutive pregnant women presenting with clinical suspicion of DVT were investigated, the diagnosis was confirmed in less than 10%,[23] compared with approximately 25% in non-pregnant women.[24]

Contrast venography is the most accurate diagnostic method for the lower limbs, but is not recommended as a first-line investigation in pregnancy, as it involves exposure of the fetus to radiation. Doppler ultrasound examination is the first-line diagnostic tool, providing 95% sensitivity and specificity for symptomatic patients.[25] A series of negative ultrasound reports together with a low level of clinical suspicion indicates that anticoagulant treatment can be discontinued or withheld. Negative ultrasound findings together with a high index of clinical suspicion indicates that further ultrasound in 1 week's time, or alternatively contrast venography, should be ordered before making any decision about the anticoagulation. If on repeat testing the diagnosis is confirmed, anticoagulation treatment should be commenced or continued. Otherwise it can be discontinued.[9] MRI of the lower limbs appears to be an accurate method for diagnosing DVT.[26] It is particularly sensitive for isolated iliac vein thrombosis, which, together with femoro-popliteal vein thrombosis, is more common in pregnancy. An example of a diagnostic algorithm for diagnosis of DVT is given in Figure 8A.1.[27]

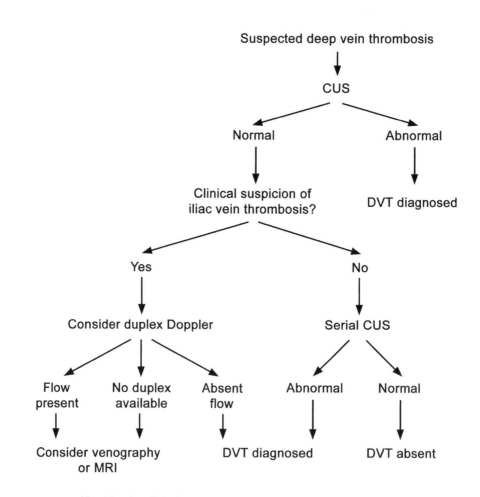

FIGURE 8A.1 Algorithm for clinically suspected DVT in pregnancy.[27] Reprinted with permission from Blackwell Publishing. DVT, deep vein thrombosis; CUS, compression ultrasonography; MRI, magnetic resonance imaging.

Pulmonary embolism (PE)

Pathophysiology

PE occurs when the clots migrate into the pulmonary circulation. Although the architecture of the microvasculature is well adapted to overcoming an obstruction, a large PE will significantly reduce left ventricular filling.

Three mechanisms are involved in the pathophysiological changes that follow PE:[28]

1   physical occlusion of the vascular system
2   platelet activation within the thrombus and subsequent release of 5-hydroxytryptamine and thromboxane A2, leading to pulmonary vasoconstriction and an increase in pulmonary vascular resistance
3   increased right ventricular afterload, which may culminate in right heart failure, causing left ventricular filling reduction and low cardiac output.

An increase in alveolar dead space, and consequently an elevated arterial/end-tidal PCO_2 gradient, are initial features. However, in awake patients hypercapnia is unusual, because hyperventilation, which might be caused by stimulation of J-receptors in the lungs or by hypoxia, is almost always present.[28]

Arterial oxygenation is also decreased. Obstruction in the pulmonary vasculature causes redistribution of pulmonary blood flow and increases the perfusion in those regions of the lung that are unaffected. If ventilation is unchanged, and blood flow increases, this results in a low ventilation/perfusion ratio in these areas. Decreased cardiac output due to right heart failure leads to decreased mixed venous oxygen saturation, exaggerating the effects of ventilation/perfusion mismatch in the lungs. Furthermore, an acute increase in right heart pressure may cause right-to-left intracardiac shunting through an unsuspected patent foramen ovale.[28]

Clinical manifestations

Clinical features indicative of PE are not specific, and depend on the severity of the obstruction, the cardiorespiratory state in general, the rate of clot fragmentation and lysis, and the presence or absence of a source for recurrent emboli.[29] Sudden onset of dyspnoea, pleuritic chest pain, non-productive cough, haemoptysis and syncope are the commonest symptoms,[22] but bronchospasm, collapse and faintness may also be suggestive of pulmonary embolism. Clinical signs associated with this condition include tachypnoea, tachycardia, arterial oxygen desaturation and raised jugular venous pressure.

The commonest ECG abnormalities are tachycardia and non-specific ST-T wave irregularities. Some of the traditional findings, such as right heart strain and acute cor pulmonale reflected in peaked P-waves in lead II (P pulmonale), right axis deviation, right bundle-branch block, an S1-Q3-T3 pattern, or atrial fibrillation, are detected in only 20% of cases. When signs and symptoms suggest PE, the absence of ECG abnormalities has a poor negative predictive value.

Some of the signs or symptoms which are suggestive of PE are regularly found during pregnancy, and must therefore be interpreted with caution. Dyspnoea, tachypnoea and chest pain are particularly common at term. This implies that a high index of suspicion is required whenever PE is suspected, and careful investigation is important.

Diagnosis

The initial diagnostic method commonly used in pregnant women with suspected PE is a ventilation/perfusion (V/Q) lung scan, which ideally should be combined with bilateral duplex ultrasound venography. A normal scan excludes the diagnosis of PE. A V/Q scan reported as suggesting medium or high probability of PE indicates that anticoagulant treatment should be commenced or continued. If the V/Q scan suggests a low probability of PE, and there is also a positive ultrasound for DVT, anticoagulant treatment should be continued. A low-risk V/Q scan and negative ultrasound venography accompanied by a high index of clinical suspicion indicates that treatment should be continued, and the test should be repeated 1 week later. If the clinical probability is still high, pulmonary angiography, MRI or helical computerised tomography should be considered. An algorithm for the diagnosis of PE is shown in Figure 8A.2.[27]

Although the chest X-ray may show elevated hemidiaphragm, atelectasis, pleural effusion or peripheral segmental or subsegmental infiltrates, it is neither specific nor sensitive. A normal chest X-ray can be seen in 25–40% of patients with PE.[30] If there

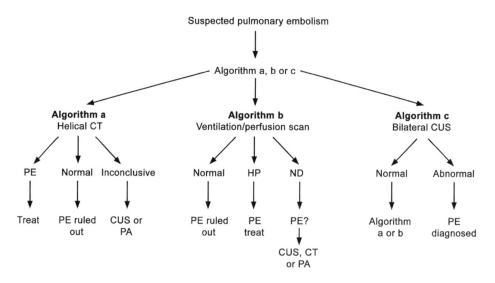

FIGURE 8A.2 Algorithm for clinically suspected pulmonary embolism in pregnancy.[27] Reprinted with permission from Blackwell Publishing. PE, pulmonary embolism; CT, computed tomography; PA, pulmonary angiography; HP, high probability; CUS, compression ultrasonography; ND, non-diagnostic result (a result that indicates an intermediate or low probability of pulmonary embolism, or that does not indicate a high probability).

is clear evidence of pulmonary pathology on the chest X-ray, an abnormal V/Q scan can be anticipated. If the cause of pathology is in doubt, one of the above imaging techniques should be used to make the diagnosis.

The radiation exposure associated with V/Q scanning, chest X-ray or limited venography is modest and unlikely to harm the fetus.[31] Therefore concerns about fetal radiation exposure should not delay the diagnostic process.

D-dimer, which is a breakdown product of fibrin, is used as a screening test for venous thromboembolism in the non-pregnant state, as it has a high negative predictive value.[32] It may be of less value in pregnancy, because it can be elevated due to the physiological changes in coagulation that occur as pregnancy progresses. It may also be increased in preterm labour, placental abruption and pre-eclampsia.[33] A more specific assay, known as the Simply RED D-dimer (SRDD) assay, together with a normal compressive ultrasonography or abnormal SRDD combined with normal serial compressive ultrasound, can safely exclude venous thromboembolism.[27,34]

Cerebral vein thrombosis

This is a less common condition in the developed world, with an incidence of approximately 1 in 10,000 deliveries and a mortality rate of less than 10%, if clinically recognised and treated.[35] The CEMD 2000–2002 report[1] cited 5 maternal deaths from cerebral vein thrombosis.

CASE 3 (1997–1999)[10]

A primigravid woman, whose mother had died of pulmonary embolism and whose father had had two strokes, booked late in pregnancy. She attended regularly and had a normal delivery at term. Eight days after delivery she developed a severe headache and became drowsy. She was admitted unconscious with a dense hemiplegia. A CT scan showed an intracerebral haematoma and thrombotic occlusion of the left transverse and sigmoid sinuses. Despite thrombolytic therapy she deteriorated and died.

Unlike PE, cerebral thrombosis may often present during hospitalisation as an inpatient. The prodromal headache has been mistaken for post-dural puncture headache, and the grand mal convulsion has been mistaken for pre-eclampsia. Obstetric anaesthetists should be alert to this condition in the differential diagnosis of headache. Contributing factors in its development are thrombophilias, including protein C and protein S deficiencies, antithrombin III deficiency, factor V Leiden, prothrombin gene mutation, hyperhomocysteinemia and antiphospholipid syndrome. Dehydration due to poor water intake may be another precipitating cause. Other causes include paroxysmal nocturnal haemoglobinuria, thrombotic thrombocytopaenic purpura, sickle-cell disease and polycythaemia.

Two possible clinical presentations depend on the initial location of the clot. In the case of cortical vein thrombosis, severe headache precedes focal or generalised convulsions, which might be followed by aphasia, weakness, focal neurological deficit and sometimes stupor. Further and faster propagation of clot through the cortical veins may be complicated by progressive neurological deficit, and even by venous infarction and intracerebral bleeding.

Thrombosis of the superior sagittal (longitudinal) sinus or the right lateral sinus is the other presentation. Headache develops due to intracranial hypertension, and clot may spread into the parasagittal motor cortex, causing lower extremity weakness and focal convulsions. If the clot spreads into the veins of the occipital complex, hemianopia and, rarely, cortical blindness may be present.

Neuroimaging studies, including CT and MRI, are the favoured diagnostic methods. If these studies fail to confirm the diagnosis, angiography (preferably digital subtraction angiography) is recommended.

The treatment of cerebral vein thrombosis includes anticoagulation and supportive measures. Heparin treatment appears to decrease the mortality rate without increasing the incidence of intracerebral haemorrhage.

Treatment of thromboembolism
Specific treatment

The specific therapy of choice in pregnant women presenting with venous thromboembolism is anticoagulation. Options for the prevention and treatment of venous thromboembolism during pregnancy and the puerperium include warfarin, unfractionated heparin (UFH), low-molecular-weight heparin (LMWH) and danaparoid sodium, a heparinoid. Hirudin, a direct thrombin inhibitor, and another heparin-like compound, fondaparinux (a pentasaccharide), which appears to have a very low rate of transplacental transfer, have not been evaluated in human pregnancy.

Warfarin, which crosses the placenta to the fetus, should be avoided during pregnancy, particularly between 6 and 12 weeks' gestation, because it is associated with an up to 5% risk of teratogenicity. In addition, it increases the risks of fetal and maternal haemorrhage (particularly at the time of delivery), neurological problems in the baby and stillbirth.[36] Although it requires close monitoring, warfarin can be safely administered to mothers after delivery and during breastfeeding, as it is not secreted in breast milk in a clinically significant amount.

UFH and LMWH do not cross the placenta, and a systematic review suggests that these agents are safe for the fetus.[37] Heparins can also be safely used during lactation, as they are not secreted in the breast milk. The regimens of administration may include continuous infusion of UFH, subcutaneous injection of UFH or subcutaneous injection of LMWH.

Intravenous UFH has been the traditional method of heparin administration in acute thromboembolic events, particularly massive PE, due to its rapid onset and the extensive experience of its use in this situation.[9] An initial intravenous bolus of 5000 IU should be given, followed by a continuous infusion of 1000–2000 IU/hour.

The treatment is usually monitored by the activated partial thromboplastin time (APTT), measured 6 hours after the loading dose, and then on a daily basis, with a therapeutic target ratio of 1.5–2.5 times the average laboratory control value.[9] The use of APTT to guide doses of UFH is not straightforward, particularly during late pregnancy. Elevated levels of factor VIII and heparin-binding plasma proteins in the pregnant woman can attenuate the response to UFH, as measured by APTT.[38] Increasing the dose of UFH to attain a 'therapeutic' APTT would be expected to result in higher heparin levels, which might increase the risk of bleeding. Therefore anti-factor Xa levels may be used to monitor heparin treatment more specifically. However, these measurements are not universally available, so the time taken to get the results is often too slow to be useful.

Subcutaneous injection of 15,000–20,000 IU of UFH twice daily, which should be given after an initial intravenous bolus of 5,000 IU, is an effective alternative to intravenous administration. A meta-analysis of randomised controlled trials showed that subcutaneous UFH was as effective, and at least as safe, as intravenous UFH in preventing recurrent venous thromboembolism in non-pregnant patients with DVT.[39]

UFH has been largely replaced by LMWH and danaparoid sodium, which are at least as effective and safe as UFH for the treatment of patients with acute proximal DVT,[40,41] and for the prevention of DVT in high-risk patients.[42] For the treatment of PE, LMWH is as effective as UFH in non-pregnant patients. Systematic reviews have concluded that LMWH is a safe alternative to UFH as an anticoagulant during pregnancy.[37] Other benefits of using LMWH include subcutaneous injection and dosing once or twice a day without the need for monitoring. This is because there is a more predictable dose response, most probably as a result of less non-specific binding to plasma heparin-binding proteins.

The biological properties of different types of LMWH are generally dependent on their molecular weight (MW) distribution, which is in the range 3,000–5,000 daltons. As the acceleration of inhibition of factor Xa (anti-Xa activity) requires only the pentasaccharide sequence (MW 1,700 daltons), and the potentiation of thrombin inhibition (anti-IIa activity) requires a minimum total chain length of 18 saccharides (MW 5,400 daltons), anti-Xa activity would be expected to exceed anti-IIa activity. The ratio of anti-Xa to anti-IIa activity varies, and the relative importance of each activity is debatable, but it is generally accepted that both types of action contribute to the anticoagulant effects of LMWH. This is why LMWH cannot be monitored with APTT. Since protamine can effectively reverse more than 90% of the anti-IIa activity and 50–70% of the anti-Xa-activity,[43] it might be possible to partially reverse the anticoagulant effect, especially in LMWH with a lower anti-Xa/anti-IIa ratio, but recommendations for routine clinical use are unavailable.

Thrombolysis using streptokinase (or urokinase) and recombinant tissue plasminogen activator might be indicated for the treatment of acute massive PE in patients who are already haemodynamically unstable.[44] However, clinical experience related to this therapeutic option is limited, and in addition there is an increased risk of major haemorrhage, particularly at term or postpartum.

Although systematic reviews suggest that some heparins are safe for the fetus,[37] several maternal complications have been described.

1   Heparin-induced osteoporosis is an important problem associated with long-term UFH use. The reported incidence of symptomatic vertebral fractures is about 2–3%, and reversible reductions in bone density have been documented in up to 30% of patients.[45] LMWH is probably associated with a lower risk of osteoporosis.[9]

2   Heparin-induced thrombocytopenia is an immune IgG-mediated reaction characterised by the development of serious, sometimes life-threatening arterial or venous thrombosis, which usually occurs between 5 and 15 days after the initial administration of heparin. It has been estimated that the risk in non-pregnant patients treated with UFH is 1–3%, but is considerably lower with LMWH.[46] In pregnant women who develop or have a history of heparin-induced thrombocytopenia, danaparoid sodium is recommended as a safe option because of the low cross-reactivity with both heparins.

Supportive measures

Supportive measures are necessary in patients who have already developed PE in order to maintain oxygenation and adequate circulation. Initial treatment may include oxygen administration and infusion of fluids and inotropes. If necessary, resuscitation should take priority over diagnostic or other therapeutic measures. Severe respiratory and circulatory compromise requires intubation, mechanical ventilation and invasive monitoring. Right atrial pressure is expected to be high, and should be maintained at a high level in an attempt to optimise the right heart cardiac output. If conventional invasive monitoring is insufficient, insertion of a pulmonary artery catheter and transoesophageal echocardiography might provide useful haemodynamic data to guide treatment.

Thromboprophylaxis

Considering only the last decade, recognition of risk factors and introduction of thromboprophylaxis have reduced the risk of postpartum death after Caesarean section, but have not yet had an impact on deaths due to antenatal thromboembolism, or to pulmonary thromboembolism following vaginal delivery. The most recent guidelines published by the Royal College of Obstetricians and Gynaecologists summarise the available evidence on prevention of venous thromboembolism during pregnancy and following vaginal delivery.[47] All of the recommendations are based on either well-controlled clinical studies or expert committee reports, and suggest that further good-quality randomised trials need to be conducted to guide prophylaxis.

CHAPTER 8B

Amniotic fluid embolism

MITKO KOCAREV AND GORDON LYONS

DEFINITION OF AMNIOTIC FLUID EMBOLISM (AFE)

AFE is an unpredictable, probably unpreventable and often rapidly progressive obstetric emergency in which amniotic fluid, fetal cells, hair or other debris enter the maternal circulation, triggering a syndrome that includes the following:

- hypoxia
- hypotension
- unconsciousness
- cardiac arrest
- coagulopathy.

In 1926, Ricardo Meyer[1] noted the presence of fetal cellular debris in the circulation of a pregnant woman following a fatal cardiovascular event. AFE was not widely recognised before 1941, when Steiner and Lushbaugh,[2] in a report on eight unexpected obstetric deaths, described material consistent with amniotic fluid debris in the pulmonary vasculature. These findings formed the basis of the earliest recognised description of the AFE syndrome.

Since these early descriptions, more than 400 cases have been documented.[3] Although most of the cases were reported during labour, sudden death in pregnancy has been attributed to AFE in various circumstances, including the following:

- during surgical termination of pregnancy
- in the second trimester[4]
- after abdominal trauma[5]
- during Caesarean section[6]
- unexpectedly postpartum.[7]

Current understanding characterises the manifestations of this condition as a multisystem reaction to toxins, rather than an embolic phenomenon.[8] This opinion is supported by strong evidence of multi-organ failure.[9] The alternative terms 'anaphylactoid syndrome in pregnancy' or 'sudden obstetric collapse syndrome' have been suggested. Over time, ideas and concepts have changed, and scepticism is necessary when considering the diagnosis of some cases attributed to AFE. However, new ideas regarding the aetiology of the condition have so far failed to reduce its incidence and severity, and it remains an important cause of maternal death.

Incidence, morbidity and mortality

There is huge variation in the reported incidence of AFE, ranging from 1 in 8,000 to 1 in 80,000 deliveries.[8] In order to accurately identify the occurrence of this condition and examine any differences or common factors between survivors and fatalities, the UK Amniotic Fluid Embolism Register was established in 1996. The entry criteria include acute hypotension or cardiac arrest, acute hypoxia, coagulopathy, absence of an alternative explanation for the observed clinical manifestation, and an onset during labour or within 30 minutes of delivery. A recent analysis from the UK Amniotic Fluid Embolism Register, which relies on voluntary reporting, gave an approximate incidence of 1 in 120,000.[10] In contrast, a population-based study from the USA reported an incidence of 1 in 20,646 live births.[7] The reasons for such variation include inaccuracies in reporting the causes of maternal death, the spectrum of the clinical presentations, lack of data on the number of non-fatal episodes, and difficulties in confirming the diagnosis.

In the UK, maternal deaths due to AFE reported over the last six CEMD reports have been just under 8% of the total number of direct deaths.[10,11] AFE has accounted for 7.5% and 10% of all maternal deaths in the USA and Australia, respectively.[12,13]

Mortality ranges from 25% in a population-based survey[7] to a maximum of 86%.[3] The most recent analysis from the UK register showed that mortality was approximately 30%.[10] The majority of deaths occur very rapidly following the acute event.[10] Disparity in these figures is probably related to the dissimilar case definitions, and to the quality of the immediate care and aftercare, which has improved with advances in intensive care.[7]

AFE is a leading cause of mortality during labour and the first few postpartum hours.[14] Among the survivors, the incidence of severe permanent neurological dysfunction is disappointingly high for a group of previously young and healthy patients. In an analysis of 46 cases of AFE from the US national registry, only 15% survived neurologically intact.[8] However, a more recent analysis from the UK register showed a substantially lower incidence of permanent neurological damage in 16% of the survivors.[10]

Risk factors

CASE 1 (1994–1996)[15]

A parous woman underwent amniocentesis because of her age. She had undergone previous instrumental deliveries due to large babies, but was persuaded to attempt a vaginal delivery. Several days after term, induction of labour was initiated with 1 mg of prostaglandin gel followed 6 hours later by 2 mg. About 3 hours later a strong contraction was noted. An epidural was set up. Fetal distress was diagnosed, and a trial of forceps was planned, but Caesarean section was performed. The baby was stillborn and was heavier than the previous babies. Severe haemorrhage occurred at operation. After some delay, hysterectomy was performed. The patient was transferred to an ICU, but died 3 days later.

This scenario strongly suggests that AFE was the cause of maternal death.

Historically, the most commonly cited risk factors associated with AFE are maternal age, multiparity, large fetus, long labour, rupture of membranes, placental abruption, uterine over-distension, use of uterine stimulants and the presence of meconium liquor. The validity of several of these factors has been brought into question as a result of the analysis from the US registry.[8] No relationship to age was found. Many clinicians believed that oxytocin use and antecedent uterine hyperstimulation increased the risk, but no relationship between the use of oxytocin and development of AFE has been established.[8] Although uterine tetany often occurs initially, it is more likely to be a response to hypoxia than to be the cause of AFE.

One factor that was consistently related to the occurrence of AFE was a tear in the fetal membranes.[8] In 78% of reported cases the signs and symptoms occurred after spontaneous or artificial rupture of the membranes, or after insertion of an intra-uterine catheter. There was also a statistically significant bias in fetal gender, the male gender being predominant. No explanation was offered for this.

The volume of amniotic material necessary to cause a recognisable clinical effect is not known. Some evidence suggests that small amounts of amniotic fluid enter the maternal circulation frequently. Squamous cells were almost universally detected from pulmonary artery catheters of pregnant women who were monitored for a variety of medical indications.[16] In contrast, an investigation in which chromium-labelled erythrocytes were injected into amniotic fluid before labour failed to detect their presence in the maternal circulation.[17]

Anyone seeking a definitive understanding is likely to be frustrated by the incomplete and often conflicting data. It seems probable that small quantities of amniotic fluid often pass into the maternal circulation, but demonstration of fetal cells is necessary to prove this. A general conclusion would be that AFE cannot be predicted or prevented.

CASE 2 (1997–1999)[18]

This patient had a termination of pregnancy under general anaesthesia in an isolated clinic. At the end of the procedure, her oxygen saturation decreased from 98% to 83% and she became bradycardic and hypotensive. She was resuscitated with adrenaline/epinephrine and was intubated and ventilated. Before transfer to the hospital, heavy vaginal blood loss was observed. Fulminant DIC became apparent. The patient developed multiple organ failure and subsequently died.

Although AFE was usually reported during labour, this case showed that it might occur in various circumstances, including surgical termination of pregnancy.

Pathophysiology

The pathophysiology is similarly unclear. The number of studies that have been designed in an attempt to develop an adequate animal model of AFE is testimony to the difficulties. In most series, an experimental injection of amniotic fluid into the animal circulation is associated with an adverse haemodynamic and/or haematological effect. It is not clear whether there are advantages to using human amniotic fluid or that of the animal under study. The problem of potential species differences exists with both approaches. Some studies have not used pregnant animals, and the importance of this is unknown. In several studies the effects of whole meconium-enriched amniotic fluid were contrasted with those of filtered amniotic fluid. Data derived from studies involving particulate-enriched amniotic fluid are considered to be irrelevant to the human population, since the concentration of particulate matter in the injectate has been many times higher than that present in human amniotic fluid, even in the presence of meconium. In primate models, an intravenous injection of autologous amniotic fluid failed to produce symptoms and signs consistent with AFE.[19] More recently, in a study of anaesthetised pregnant goats using homologous amniotic fluid, haemodynamic alterations and clinical findings similar to those seen in women have been observed.[20] These reactions were particularly pronounced when the injectate included meconium.

The outcome of the studies is neither consistent nor conclusive. We are left to depend on numerous case reports involving pregnant women with AFE to provide additional information about the pathophysiology.

When clinical data collected during the resuscitation of several parturients are evaluated, a biphasic response to this condition becomes apparent. The initial response of the pulmonary vasculature to the presence of amniotic fluid is vasospasm, producing a transient but intense increase in pulmonary artery pressure. This may account for the development of right heart failure, which is often fatal. Low cardiac output leads to increased ventilation/perfusion mismatch, hypoxia and hypotension. The transient nature of this initial haemodynamic response, which lasts for not more than 30 minutes, could account for the lack of evidence relating to pulmonary hypertension in humans, as all reported human data were collected at least 70 minutes after initial symptoms. Support for this response is found in animal models, where infusion of amniotic fluid into the circulation produces an immediate significant increase in pulmonary artery resistance and mean pulmonary artery pressure, which returns to baseline levels within 10–30 minutes after injection.[21,22] In addition, reports of transoesophageal echocardiography, which was performed in pregnant women within 15 minutes after the onset of the symptoms of AFE, confirmed the occurrence of acute severe pulmonary hypertension and massive right heart failure.[23,24]

Women who survive the initial events may enter a second phase of haemodynamic compromise, primarily involving left ventricular failure and pulmonary oedema with return of normal right heart function. Data from invasive haemodynamic monitoring of affected patients are consistent with the occurrence of left ventricular dysfunction. The mechanism of left ventricular failure is uncertain. Animal data suggest the presence of possible coronary artery spasm and myocardial ischaemia.[25] The hypoxia associated with AFE could lead to left ventricular dysfunction, although the possibility of a direct myocardial depressant effect cannot be excluded.

Many authors have suggested that humoral factors mediated by prostaglandins and other arachidonic acid metabolites might contribute to the haemodynamic changes associated with AFE. One animal model showed that $PGF_{2\alpha}$ and amniotic fluid from labouring women, in contrast to the fluid of non-labouring women, produced hypotension and elevated CVP when injected into cats.[26] Another study demonstrated that pre-treatment of rats with an inhibitor of leucotriene synthesis overcame the fatal haemodynamic collapse observed following experimental AFE in this species.[27] There is evidence that the concentration of prostaglandins PGE_2 and $PGF_{2\alpha}$ in the amniotic fluid increases as the pregnancy progresses, reaching a dramatic peak during labour.[28] Unstable products of the prostaglandin synthetase enzyme complex in the amniotic fluid might, theoretically, be converted to thromboxane, prostaglandin or prostacycline, which are vasoactive substances. Moreover, in two cases of AFE, intense expression of endothelin-1 was observed in the amniotic squames.[29] Since endothelin is a potent vasoconstrictor and bronchoconstrictor, this could account for the early and transient haemodynamic alteration of pulmonary hypertension seen in this syndrome.

These considerations suggest that it is the chemical composition rather than the volume of amniotic fluid that is responsible for the haemodynamic effects.

In addition to hypotension and pulmonary oedema, which might be cardiogenic or inflammatory in origin, as many as 40% of patients who survive the initial event may develop a secondary coagulopathy and haemorrhage.[8] In some women, this may be the first and only clinical manifestation. The aetiology of the coagulopathy is unclear. Although clear amniotic fluid has been shown to have direct factor-X-activating properties, the amount of procoagulant is not sufficient to cause significant clinical intravascular coagulation.[30] Some *in-vitro* studies with amniotic fluid have found a thromboplastin-like effect, with shortened whole blood clotting time, induction of platelet aggregation, release of platelet factor III and activation of the complement cascade.[31] A more recent study of tissue factor and tissue factor pathway inhibitor showed that levels were 44 times higher in amniotic fluid than in plasma, and lower levels of tissue factor pathway inhibitor were found in the plasma of pregnant women than in that of non-pregnant women.[32] This may explain why the presence of amniotic fluid in the maternal circulation triggers intravascular coagulation and consumptive coagulopathy.

Clinical features

The symptoms and signs associated with AFE are non-specific, and include the following:

- acute shortness of breath
- severe hypotension
- cardiovascular collapse
- cyanosis
- cardiac dysrhythmias
- coma
- an absence of any other explanation for the event
- onset during delivery or within 30 minutes of delivery or abortion
- consumptive coagulopathy in > 80% of cases.[8]

It is becoming increasingly clear that the presentation might be more subtle, and that subclinical and atypical events might initially be unrecognised. In 10–20% of cases the presenting symptoms may be maternal convulsions or haemorrhage.[33] Sudden fetal bradycardia followed by coagulopathy, despite adequate maternal cardiopulmonary status, should raise the possibility of AFE.[34] The lack of specificity with regard to presentation means that it is essential to maintain a high index of suspicion for AFE whenever a mother or fetus becomes unwell at delivery whether in early or late pregnancy.

Diagnosis

CASE 3 (2000–2002)[11]

A mother had been normotensive throughout a normal pregnancy and had a spontaneous labour with a retained placenta. She then complained of central chest pain and was given oxygen. However, a short while later, prior to induction of anaesthesia for the removal of the placenta, her blood pressure was elevated and she had a grand mal seizure. The diagnosis was considered to be amniotic fluid embolus or pulmonary embolus, and the patient was transferred to the intensive-care unit. It was noted that her platelets and fibrinogen levels had fallen, and at this stage she had massive vaginal bleeding. Despite a subtotal hysterectomy and massive transfusion of blood and blood products, she had a cardiac arrest from which she could not be resuscitated. The autopsy was detailed and thorough. In particular, multiple blocks of lung were stained immunocytochemically for fetal squames with the antibody LP34, and were also stained for fetal mucin. These results were also reviewed and repeated by the local pathology assessor, and were again negative. In addition, histology of the uterine bed showed the features of an acute atherosclerosis which, although not diagnostic, are typical of pre-eclamptic change.

This case illustrates the difficulties involved in the accurate diagnosis of AFE, and it emphasises the need for detailed analysis of maternal death. There is no routine diagnostic procedure for confirming the occurrence of AFE.

The finding of squamous cells and other debris of presumed fetal origin in maternal pulmonary vasculature, once considered pathognomonic, is now known to be neither specific nor sensitive. Only 50% of patients who are resuscitated from AFE have these as positive findings.[8] Although detection of squamous cells has commonly been confirmed in the maternal pulmonary circulation of women undergoing pulmonary artery catheterisation, these cells might be due to epidermal contamination following venepuncture.[16] It has not proved possible histologically to differentiate between adult and fetal squames.

To overcome this uncertainty, various diagnostic stains have been investigated. One study demonstrated that fetal mucin could be identified in the pulmonary vasculature using the monoclonal antibody TKH-2.[35] TKH-2 immunostaining appears to be a sensitive method of detecting mucin in the lungs of affected patients. Another study, which measured the plasma concentration of zinc coproporphyrine, which is a characteristic component of meconium, found a higher concentration of this substance in patients with AFE and those with AFE-like symptoms.[36] Clinical experience of the use of both of these methods is too limited for any recommendations to be made, but it may become possible to distinguish between maternal and fetal tissue debris.

In approaching AFE as an anaphylactic reaction, a number of reports have described increased levels of serum tryptase.[37,38] However, a recent series of nine cases demonstrated normal tryptase levels with a low complement.[39] These findings suggest that complement activation rather than mast-cell degranulation might play a role in AFE.[40]

In addition to the clinical features of AFE, certain tests and methods may help to diagnose the condition. Chest X-ray is usually non-specific, but evidence of pulmonary oedema, enlarged heart and pleural effusion might be seen. A 12-lead ECG may show tachycardia, ST-segment and T-wave changes, and findings consistent with right ventricular strain. Echocardiography can estimate pulmonary pressures and confirm severe acute right or left ventricular failure. A lung V/Q scan may aid the diagnosis of AFE, and show non-specific multiple perfusion defects. Blood and clotting series can show changes consistent with coagulopathy.

Post-mortem diagnosis may be aided by the detection of fetal debris in the pulmonary vasculature. However, if the patient survives for several days, any sign of fetal debris may be lost.

The differential diagnosis includes the following:

- septic shock
- aspiration pneumonitis
- acute myocardial infarction
- pulmonary thromboembolism
- venous air embolism
- anaphylaxis
- obstetric complications (placental abruption, uterine rupture, eclampsia)
- anaesthetic complication (total spinal anaesthesia or systemic local anaesthetic toxicity).

Management

The management of AFE is supportive and directed towards the maintenance of oxygenation, cardiac output and blood pressure, and correction of the coagulopathy. If the clinical situation requires it, full cardiopulmonary resuscitation must be initiated. Earlier recommendations to treat initial pulmonary hypertension and acute right heart failure with a vasodilator are not applicable in situations where patients are hypotensive. Treatment should be directed towards oxygenation, increasing cardiac output and maintaining the blood pressure. Prompt and aggressive support may decrease the severity of neurological sequelae and prevent multiple organ failure.

Delivery of the fetus by Caesarean section must be initiated as soon as possible.[8]

Uterine tone may need to be re-established with bimanual massage, uterine packing and oxytocin or prostaglandin analogues.[3] Improvement in cardiac output and consequently in uterine perfusion facilitates uterine muscle tone.

Invasive central haemodynamic monitoring, including a pulmonary artery catheter, provides critical information and guides specific treatment. Optimisation of preload with rapid volume infusion is imperative, and adequate inotropic support with adrenaline, dopamine or dobutamine must be provided. Transthoracic or transoesophageal echocardiography may guide fluid therapy with evaluation of left ventricular filling. After oxygenation, correction and optimisation of cardiac output, fluid therapy should be restricted to maintenance levels to prevent the development of pulmonary oedema and subsequent ARDS.

The treatment of coagulopathy should be guided by the coagulation profile. Component therapy is often successful. Therapeutic heparinisation to limit the intravascular coagulation and consumptive coagulopathy is not routinely recommended. If an epidural catheter is inserted before the onset of AFE, it should be removed as soon as the normal coagulation profile has been restored.[41] Peripheral neurological function should be assessed frequently, to allow early detection of epidural haematoma.

Future pregnancies

Two cases of successful pregnancy outcomes in women who survived AFE during earlier pregnancies have been reported.[42] This supports the role of qualitatively abnormal amniotic fluid in the pathogenesis of this condition, which might be different in subsequent pregnancy. Repeated AFE is probably an unlikely event.

CHAPTER 9

Sepsis

MICHELLE HAYES

In the UK, the incidence of severe sepsis in adult intensive-care units is 27.7%, which amounts to about 23,211 cases per year.[1] The hospital mortality rate is 44.7%, which means that there are an estimated 10,375 deaths per year.[1] In the obstetric population, severe sepsis was a significant contributor to maternal mortality until 1935, when the introduction of Prontosil, followed by sulphonamides and penicillin in the following decade, caused it to fall. Sepsis is now an infrequent but nevertheless important contributor to maternal mortality. In the most recent CEMD report (2000–2002) there were 13 deaths due to genital tract sepsis and 14 deaths due to non-obstetric-related sepsis.[2] This chapter looks at the historical and pathophysiological aspects of severe sepsis, together with its clinical presentation. It also looks at the lessons that can be learned from maternal deaths due to severe sepsis, and reviews recent guidelines for management of these patients.[3]

Historical aspect

Sepsis is among the leading causes of preventable maternal death not only in developing countries, but in developed countries as well. It is interesting that as far back as 1795, Alexander Gordon expressed the opinion that birth attendants carried the infection during the outbreak of puerperal fever in Aberdeen. This mode of transmission was confirmed later by others, and most famously by Oliver Wendell Holmes in the USA in 1841. In 1846, Ignaz Phillip Semmelweis was working in the obstetric department of the General Hospital in Vienna. He noticed that in one ward attended by medical students, puerperal fever was very common and the mortality rate was 29%. However, in another ward, which was attended by midwifery pupils, the mortality rate was only 3%. He hypothesised that the disease was carried by the hands of medical students and physicians who had previously been in the post-mortem room. In May 1847, Semmelweis ordered hand washing with chlorinated water before deliveries, and the mortality rate plummeted. Unfortunately, Semmelweis found that his conclusions did not receive immediate acclaim from his colleagues and superiors. Although some of them recognised the importance of his discovery, there were many in Vienna who rejected his theories and treated them with scepticism and ridicule. In 1849 he moved on to work in Hungary. However, his final years were plagued by psychiatric illness, and he died in 1865 in a psychiatric hospital from septic shock as a result of an infected wound of his middle finger.[4] Paradoxically, within a few years of his death the use of antiseptics and the principles of asepsis began to be accepted. The introduction in 1935 of an effective treatment in the form of antibiotics (sulphonamides and penicillin) resulted in a rapid fall in the number of maternal deaths. However, as deaths from other direct causes fell, sepsis as a result of septic abortion again emerged as a leading cause of death. Since the Abortion Act was passed in 1967 there have been only 146 direct deaths associated with septic abortion. In fact, in the CEMD 1982–1984 report,[5] no deaths could be directly attributed to puerperal sepsis. Unfortunately, in subsequent reports, mortality rates have increased again (*see* Table 9.1).[6–10]

TABLE 9.1   Numbers of direct deaths associated with genital tract sepsis and mortality rate per million maternities in the UK, for the period 1985–2002

TRIENNIUM	SEPSIS IN EARLY PREGNANCY*	PUERPERAL SEPSIS	SEPSIS AFTER SURGICAL PROCEDURES	SEPSIS BEFORE OR DURING LABOUR	TOTAL	RATE PER MILLION MATERNITIES
1985–87[10]	3	2	2	2	9	4.0
1988–90[9]	8	4	5	0	17	7.2
1991–93[8]	4	4	5	2	15	6.5
1994–96[7]	2	11	3	1	17	7.3
1997–99[6]	6	4	1	7	18	8.5
2000–02[2]	4	5	3	1	13	6.5

*Early pregnancy includes deaths following miscarriage, ectopic and other causes.

Pathophysiology

Sepsis is defined as a systemic inflammatory response to infection, and severe sepsis has an associated organ dysfunction.[11] Septic shock is defined as sepsis with hypotension that is refractory to fluid resuscitation.[11]

Evolving inflammatory responses can trigger pathophysiological changes that lead to severe sepsis. In severe sepsis, microbial products such as the cell wall components of Gram-positive bacteria and the outer cell membrane of Gram-negative bacteria bind to binding proteins which are recognised by CD14 receptors on the surface of immune cells.[12,13] These immune cells, principally monocytes/macrophages and polymorphonuclear neutrophils, are not only able to recognise the pathogenic agents and their products so that they can phagocytose and destroy them, but can also release mediators that can activate other cells.[14,15] These mediators include potent anti-inflammatory cytokines such as tumour necrosis factor (TNF), interleukin 1 (IL1), interleukin 6 (IL6) and interleukin 8 (IL8). These can combine with other cells, leading to the release of adhesion molecules, metabolites of arachidonic acid pathways, and products of leucocytes, platelets and vessel walls. In addition, the coagulation, complement and kinin systems are all activated.

The inflammatory process is tightly regulated and functions to confine the spread of infection locally, and it is clear that not all cases of bacteraemia or sepsis progress to severe sepsis or septic shock. When they do progress, there are serious effects on the cardiovascular system. The systemic vascular resistance decreases, often to a quarter of its normal value, which results in hypotension despite a normal or elevated cardiac output.[16] The vasodilatation is thought to be due to the production of nitric oxide (NO) by the endothelium. NO is produced from L-arginine by nitric oxide synthase, and it directly relaxes the smooth muscle in blood vessels. There are two different forms, namely the constitutional form and the inducible form (iNOS). In sepsis, iNOS expression is stimulated by cytokines such as IL1 and TNFα.[17] This is followed by massive NO production and profound vasodilatation. Myocardial function is also depressed, with decreased myocardial contractility accompanied by dilatation of the ventricle.[18,19] These patients therefore require greater cardiac filling pressures than non-septic patients. In time, the patient may also become unresponsive to catecholamines, which may be due in part to adrenocortical suppression.[20]

In pregnancy, the normal cardiovascular changes that occur are similar to those that occur in sepsis in that there is vasodilatation and an increased cardiac output with tachycardia. The blood pressure is maintained by the augmented cardiac output. Further vasodilatation as a result of sepsis together with myocardial dysfunction can compromise both the maternal and uteroplacental circulation.

Sepsis is also accompanied by activation of the coagulation cascade via tissue factor- and factor VII-dependent generation of thrombin. Tissue factor is capable of activating factor VII, which activates further steps in the extrinsic coagulation pathway. Further thrombin production is then maintained by the intrinsic pathway. This leads to the development of disseminated intravascular coagulation (DIC). Activated protein C, its cofactor protein S, thrombomodulin and antithrombin III are natural anticoagulants, and they provide a negative feedback mechanism for the coagulation cascade. However, the concentrations of protein C and antithrombin III are reduced in sepsis.[21,22] The net effect is a procoagulant state. The situation may be exacerbated during pregnancy because the latter is also associated with a hypercoagulable state. The formation of emboli in the microvasculature is thought to lead to microcirculatory dysfunction and ultimately organ failure. It may also lead to pregnancy loss and maternal death.

Clinical presentation of severe sepsis

In early sepsis, low blood pressure and high heart rate are associated with a high cardiac output and a low peripheral vascular resistance, with warm peripheries and bounding pulses. In contrast, late sepsis presents with a low cardiac output and high systemic vascular resistance – these patients are peripherally cold, sweaty, have weak, thready pulses and need urgent resuscitation. It is important to take into account the fact that the normal physiological changes of pregnancy include tachycardia, vasodilatation and a raised cardiac output, and these changes will increase even further with sepsis. Although pulmonary pressures remain within normal limits during pregnancy, pregnant patients are at greater risk of developing pulmonary oedema due to pregnancy-induced decreases in colloid osmotic pressure.[23] The increase in microvascular permeability due to the release of inflammatory mediators during sepsis will put them at further risk. As sepsis progresses, there will be reduced uterine perfusion and reduced fetal oxygenation, and a fetal acidosis will develop. In addition, maternal dyspnoea may be secondary to normal physiological changes in pregnancy. However, a patient with this symptom warrants prompt evaluation, as it may be due to severe sepsis. Other manifestations of severe sepsis include a high, normal or low temperature, hypothermia being associated with higher mortality rates.[24] An increased white cell count is common, although it can be depressed. The ESR and CRP may be raised. Severe sepsis is also typically associated with increased lactate levels (> 2 mmol/litre), and insulin requirements may also increase. Oliguria is often present, and the patient may be confused, agitated or drowsy. In addition, there may be cutaneous and ophthalmological manifestations.

Genital tract sepsis

Deaths due to sepsis in the obstetric population can be classified as direct or indirect. Direct deaths are secondary to genital tract infection and indirect deaths are due to non-obstetric-related infections and mastitis. In the CEMD reports, deaths due to puerperal sepsis are classified as those following vaginal delivery. Other deaths are subdivided into those following sepsis in early pregnancy, sepsis after surgical procedures and sepsis before or during labour (*see* Table 9.1).

Genital tract sepsis may be a consequence of postpartum endometritis, septic abortion, intra-amniotic infection, septic thrombophlebitis or wound infection. Patients may be at greater risk of infection if they have comorbidity, such as diabetes or HIV-related disease.

Postpartum endometritis is caused by an infection of the decidua with extension to the myometrium and parametrial tissues, and is usually caused by a mixture of aerobic and anaerobic organisms. Risk factors for infection include chorioamnionitis, prolonged rupture of membranes, premature labour, multiple vaginal examinations, retained products of conception and Caesarean section. The frequency of endometritis in women who undergo a vaginal delivery is approximately 1–3%. However, in women who have an elective Caesarean section this figure is around 5–15%, but it can be as high as 35%, depending on the particular situation. The use of prophylactic antibiotics has been shown to reduce this rate of infection.[25] With regard to the choice of antibiotic, both ampicillin and first-generation cephalosporins have been shown to have similar efficacy.[26] Septic abortion is an infection following a termination of pregnancy (either spontaneous or induced). The risk of infection following an induced abortion is about 1%. Infections can range from localised infection to the formation of a pelvic abscess. Intra-amniotic infections include a spectrum of diseases such as chorioamnionitis, amnionitis and amniotic fluid infection. Intra-amniotic infections can complicate up to 10% of deliveries.[27] Sepsis complicates intra-amniotic infection in 0.5–1.3% of cases.[28] Septic pelvic thrombophlebitis can also be a cause of puerperal fever, and is thought to follow pelvic infection. Patients present with a fever that is unresponsive to antibiotics, and the diagnosis is confirmed clinically or radiologically. The condition responds rapidly to intravenous heparin. Wounds are also at risk of infection, and patients who are particularly susceptible include those who have had a Caesarean section, those with drains or haematomas, and those with obesity and diabetes. The most severe of these infections is necrotising fasciitis, which has a significant mortality rate.[29]

In septic obstetric patients, the commonest causative organisms are endotoxin-producing aerobic Gram-negative rods, followed by Gram-positive bacteria and mixed or fungal infections. Beta-haemolytic streptococcus Group A was a major cause of puerperal sepsis in the nineteenth century and the first half of the twentieth century. Although the incidence declined following the introduction of effective antibiotics, it remains an important cause of sepsis.

Direct deaths associated with genital tract sepsis

In many of the cases reported, sepsis appears to have been so overwhelming that it is unclear whether much could have been done to change the course of events. However, there are lessons to learn with regard to prevention, education, communication, detection and treatment. The following are some of the case studies taken from the last four CEMD reports (covering the period 1991–2002) that demonstrate areas of management that could be improved upon.

CASE 1 (1991–1993)[8]

A parous woman had a raised alpha-fetoprotein level at 13 weeks' gestation, and an ultrasound scan at 17 weeks confirmed that the fetus was abnormal. She was offered termination of the pregnancy, but declined. She was admitted to hospital at 28 weeks with spontaneous rupture of the membranes, refused induction, and was treated conservatively without antibiotic cover. Four days later she developed rigors and lower abdominal pain. There was an associated intrauterine death. She was commenced on antibiotics. Induction of labour with prostaglandins was attempted, but failed. A clotting screen disclosed a developing coagulopathy, and it was decided to deliver the patient by Caesarean section. Prior to the operation the patient collapsed, but a general anaesthetic was administered, following which she had a cardiac arrest. Despite intensive resuscitation measures she did not recover. The autopsy confirmed that the cause of death was septicaemia due to chorioamnionitis. Culture showed a mixed growth of *Proteus* and coliform organisms. The stillborn infant had multiple congenital abnormalities.

LESSONS

- Staff must be aware of the risk factors for infection, and understand that repeated screening for infection is vital.
- Early recognition of severe sepsis is important, so that treatment can be instituted as soon as possible.
- If a patient is going to theatre for a surgical procedure, they must be adequately resuscitated prior to general anaesthesia. These patients are already tachycardic and vasodilated as a result of the normal physiological changes of pregnancy, and they will be further vasodilated by severe sepsis. Any further vasodilatation as a result of an anaesthetic agent may cause rapid decompensation with a significant decrease in cardiac output and hypotension leading to cardiac arrest.

CASE 2 (1994–1996)[7]

A young parous woman had a planned home confinement with an uncomplicated labour and delivery at 39 weeks' gestation, supervised by a midwife. Postnatal observations were satisfactory for 4 days. She then had an isolated episode of severe diarrhoea for which she received treatment after contact with a locum GP. She was seen by the midwife the next day, and on examination her temperature was 40°C and her pulse rate was 140 beats/min. The lochia were normal and not offensive, and there was no abdominal tenderness. The midwife contacted the GP, who attended the patient and after an examination said that he considered her condition to be satisfactory. However, he failed to record her temperature. When the midwife revisited the patient later the same day, her temperature and pulse remained elevated. The next morning the patient's husband called an ambulance as her condition had suddenly deteriorated. She died soon afterwards. An autopsy confirmed that she had died from group A beta-haemolytic streptococcus.

LESSONS

- A temperature of 40°C with a tachycardia of 140 beats/min is a manifestation of severe sepsis. Therefore the patient requires urgent assessment in hospital.
- Diarrhoea can be a sign of intra-abdominal or pelvic sepsis.
- All members of the multi-disciplinary team that may be looking after a pregnant woman need to be able to recognise an individual who is sick.

CASE 3 (1994–1996)[7]

A primigravida had an uneventful pregnancy and was admitted in spontaneous labour at 38 weeks' gestation. She was delivered by ventouse extraction because of fetal distress in the late second stage of labour. The immediate postnatal period was uneventful, but on the second day after delivery she complained of abdominal pain. She was apyrexial, but her pulse was 100 beats/min. On the following day she remained apyrexial but complained of increasing abdominal pain. The episiotomy scar was reddened and the lochia were offensive. A vaginal swab revealed a strong growth of beta-haemolytic streptococci. The patient rapidly developed septic shock, and a total abdominal hysterectomy and vulval debridement were performed. Despite intensive therapy, including hyperbaric oxygen, the woman's condition slowly deteriorated with multiple organ failure. She died 6 weeks after delivery.

LESSONS

- Severe postnatal infections can have a rapid onset, and if not recognised may be fatal. Therefore all staff must be aware of the clinical features of severe sepsis. These include tachycardia and tachypnoea, and although these can be normal physiological changes, the patient must be assessed as soon as possible.
- Antibiotics must be administered within the first hour of recognition of severe sepsis, after appropriate cultures have been obtained. To optimise identification of causative organisms, at least two blood cultures should be obtained. Cultures from other appropriate sites should also be obtained (e.g. urine, CSF, wounds, respiratory secretions or other body fluids).[3]

CASE 4 (1997–1999)[6]

An older parous woman with a multiple pregnancy had normal progress until late in pregnancy, when she was referred to hospital with a brief history of vomiting and rigors. On admission, she showed classical signs of septicaemia with extreme hypotension. There was no uterine tenderness, but the fetuses were dead. Active resuscitation was undertaken and the patient was commenced on broad-spectrum antibiotics.

An artificial rupture of the membranes was performed and oxytocin was commenced. The patient then developed DIC and severe vaginal bleeding. A Caesarean section was performed because of the deterioration in her condition. She had further vaginal bleeding, and an unsuccessful attempt was made to treat this by arterial embolisation. The patient was given large quantities of blood, plasma and platelets throughout. There was a significant delay of around 2 to 3 hours in obtaining platelets, as they had to come from the blood transfusion service many miles away. Blood cultures reported group A haemolytic streptococcus. The patient developed multiple organ failure and died a few days postpartum. Because it had been stated that this woman was allergic to penicillin, she was not given the antibiotic on admission. When the culture confirmed that the organism responsible for the infection was a streptococcus, a test dose of penicillin gave no reaction, and she was then started on this antibiotic. A post-mortem was not performed.

LESSONS

- Antibiotics must be administered within the first hour of recognition of severe sepsis, as soon as appropriate cultures have been obtained. To optimise identification of causative organisms, at least two blood cultures should be obtained. Cultures from other appropriate sites should also be obtained (e.g. urine, CSF, wounds, sputum or other body fluids).[3]
- Early discussion of antibiotic therapy with microbiologists is essential. The choice of drugs should be guided by the susceptibility patterns of micro-organisms in the community and in the hospital.[3] The basis on which allergy has been diagnosed should be elucidated, as in many cases it is not true allergy.

CASE 5 (1997–1999)[6]

A parous woman was admitted to hospital with spontaneous rupture of the membranes at 30 weeks' gestation. A sepsis screen was negative on admission. Twenty-four hours later the patient developed tachycardia, pyrexia and intrauterine death. A short time afterwards she had rigors and was transferred to the labour ward, where intravenous antibiotics were commenced. A vaginal examination confirmed that she was in labour, and an epidural was sited. Approximately 1 hour later her condition rapidly deteriorated, with pulmonary oedema and hypotension. She required intubation due to breathing difficulties, and developed DIC shortly after delivery, when her blood pressure was unrecordable. Despite active resuscitation, she died within the hour. An autopsy confirmed that death was due to *E. coli* septicaemia following chorioamnionitis.

LESSONS

- Antibiotics must be administered within the first hour of recognition of severe sepsis.
- To site an epidural under these circumstances appears inappropriate. It would have resulted in further vasodilatation in an already compromised patient. Furthermore, any damage to an epidural vein during insertion would provide a focus for development of an epidural abscess.
- This patient became seriously ill very rapidly. Therefore the critical care outreach or the intensive-care team should have been involved at an early stage.

CASE 6 (1997–1999)[6]

An older multigravid woman, with a history of poor attendance at antenatal clinics, was admitted to a DGH in mid-pregnancy with a 5-day history of passing fluid per vaginum and severe suprapubic pain. The diagnosis of ruptured membranes was not confirmed on examination, and she was discharged home within 24 hours on oral antibiotics. She was readmitted the next day with obvious ruptured membranes, and was transferred to a teaching hospital with neonatal ICU facilities. Within 48 hours she was pyrexial with a tachycardia and complaining of abdominal pain. Intravenous antibiotics were commenced and she delivered a stillborn infant. A general anaesthetic was administered shortly afterwards for removal of a retained placenta. It proved impossible to extubate her following the general anaesthetic, and she was transferred to the ICU with established ARDS. She remained critically ill, and 2 days after delivery a hysterectomy was performed to eliminate a possible focus of infection in the uterus. The patient's condition did not improve during the next few weeks in the ICU, and she died from multiple organ failure. An autopsy showed infection with *Klebsiella*, but this was probably acquired in the ICU, and the underlying cause of death was most probably Gram-negative bacillary septicaemia, secondary to intrauterine infection.

LESSONS

- This patient clearly had risk factors for infection.
- Pyrexia, tachycardia and abdominal pain are features of severe sepsis.
- Antibiotics should be administered within the first hour of recognition of severe sepsis, after consultation with the microbiologists.

CASE 7 (1997–1999)[6]

A parous woman had a history of previous Caesarean sections, including one with abnormal adherence of the placenta. In this pregnancy she had a known placenta praevia, and an emergency Caesarean section was performed under regional anaesthesia by a middle-grade doctor without consultant involvement. There was excessive blood loss during the operation, and the uterus was closed with placental tissue *in situ*. Transfusion with 4 units of blood resulted in a haemoglobin level of only 7.1 g/dl. There was no record of antibiotics having been administered. The patient was discharged from hospital a week later, and was readmitted with vaginal bleeding and pyrexia a few days after this. She developed septicaemia and DIC and had further operations to control the bleeding, without success. She died 3 weeks postpartum from multiple organ failure. *Streptococcus faecalis* was isolated from high vaginal swabs and blood culture. Histology confirmed a placenta accreta.

LESSONS

- When a patient is high risk, it is vitally important to involve senior staff in their care from an early stage, and even more so if there are problems at surgery.
- Antibiotics did not appear to have been given in this case. Data from the Cochrane Library support the use of prophylactic antibiotics during Caesarean section.[25]

CASE 8 (2000–2002)[2]

A woman with a history of 'panic attacks' developed a persistent tachycardia (130–170 beats/min) after delivery, and her increasingly bizarre behaviour was repeatedly attributed to a psychiatric cause, without either further investigation or seeking consultant advice. She was admitted to a psychiatric hospital, but was then quickly transferred to the local general hospital, where she died shortly after arrival. Autopsy revealed an infected necrotic uterus, and several different organisms (streptococcus groups B and D, *Staphylococcus aureus*, *Bacteroides*, *E. coli*, Gram-positive rods) were identified in the uterus, blood and gastrointestinal tract. There was also marked left ventricular hypertrophy, which probably accounted for some of her symptoms and was probably due to a peripartum cardiomyopathy, although histological examination was not performed to confirm this.

LESSONS

- In this case it is important to realise that extreme tachycardia is rarely a result of anxiety, but if it is, it should settle with reassurance. Other causes should have been considered, such as infection and cardiac abnormalities.

CASE 9 (2000–2002)[2]

This woman delivered in water with faecal contamination, and became unwell with a temperature of 40° C, pain and infection in her buttock and leg. She developed overwhelming sepsis and died despite intensive medical and surgical treatment.

In another case, community carers were unaware of a history of ragged membranes, and did not immediately suspect sepsis in a recently delivered woman.

LESSONS

- Communication about risk factors for infection is of paramount importance.

Indirect deaths due to non-obstetric-related sepsis

It is important to remember that pregnant women and women in the postpartum period are also at risk of other infections outside the genital tract, and to be aware of the morbidity and mortality associated with these infections. They include mastitis and other non-obstetric causes of sepsis, such as urinary tract infections, pneumonia, meningitis, intra-abdominal infections, hepatitis, HIV, malaria, Lyme disease, herpetic disease, listeriosis, *Mycobacterium tuberculosis* and toxoplasmosis. The numbers of these deaths, for the last four triennia, are shown in Table 9.2. During pregnancy, women may be at increased risk of pneumonia due to elevation of the diaphragm by the uterus and delayed gastric emptying. They may also have a weaker cough. In addition, there may be an increased risk of pyelonephritis due to a reduction in renal concentrating ability, smooth muscle relaxation with ureteral dilatation, bladder flaccidity and vesico-ureteral reflux.[30]

TABLE 9.2   Numbers of deaths due to non-obstetric-related sepsis

TRIENNIUM	NUMBER OF DEATHS
1991–93[8]	8
1994–96[7]	9
1997–99[6]	13
2000–02[2]	14

CASE 10 (1991–1993)[8]

A patient was admitted in the late afternoon feeling cold and shivery with backache. She developed a fever of 39°C with severe vomiting and diarrhoea during the night. Intrauterine fetal death occurred. Later that morning antibiotics were started, but she rapidly developed DIC, and could not be resuscitated following a cardiac arrest 2 hours later. Blood cultures yielded pure profuse growth of group A beta-haemolytic streptococcus.

LESSONS

- This patient demonstrated signs of severe sepsis from admission. Diarrhoea and vomiting can also be manifestations of this.
- Antibiotics should have been administered on admission.
- Group A beta-haemolytic streptococcus is still an important cause of sepsis.

CASE 11 (1991–1993)[8]

This patient was 34 weeks pregnant when she suddenly developed vomiting and abdominal pain one night. Over the past week other members of the family had suffered symptoms of upper respiratory tract infection. By early in the morning the woman was complaining of shortness of breath, and the pain was more severe. While arrangements were being made for her admission to the maternity unit she had a respiratory arrest from which she could not be resuscitated. At autopsy she was found to have DIC. Gram-positive organisms were seen on histology, and group A beta-haemolytic streptococcus was isolated from all swabs taken post-mortem, including vaginal swabs. The portal of entry could have been the nasopharynx or possibly the genital tract.

LESSONS

- Once again abdominal pain and vomiting may be signs of severe sepsis.
- Group A beta-haemolytic streptococcus is still an important cause of infection.

CASE 12 (1994–1996)[7]

A young woman became ill in the latter half of her pregnancy. She initially called her GP, who diagnosed a flu-like illness, and when her condition deteriorated she was admitted to the labour ward of a consultant unit. There she was found to be short of breath with headache, blurred vision and fever. She had a purpuric rash all over her body. Intrauterine death was diagnosed by ultrasound. The patient was seen by obstetric and medical registrars, who noted cyanosis and the worsening rash. She was initially thought to have a pulmonary embolism or overwhelming sepsis with DIC. The intensive-care-unit registrar thought that the very high levels of fibrin degradation products were due to DIC secondary to intrauterine death. The patient was transferred to an intensive-care unit and died very soon afterwards. Blood cultures later confirmed meningococcal septicaemia.

LESSONS

- A purpuric rash is a classic feature of meningococcal septicaemia.
- Antibiotics and resuscitation should have been started immediately on presentation, as these patients deteriorate extremely rapidly.
- Senior help should be called for immediately.

CASE 13 (1994–1996)[7]

A young woman contracted chicken pox from a child. She presented to her GP with varicella rash at 28 weeks' gestation and was treated symptomatically. Two days later she was admitted to hospital because she had developed breathlessness, vomiting and dehydration. Pneumonitis was diagnosed and acyclovir was given. She rapidly deteriorated, despite intensive care. The fetus died, and 5 days after admission it was decided to deliver her in the hope that this would improve matters, but she died during the Caesarian section. Autopsy confirmed varicella pneumonia.

LESSONS

- Acyclovir should have been given when this patient first presented to her GP.[31]
- The fact that she died in theatre suggests that she may have required further resuscitation prior to transfer.

CASE 14 (1997–1999)[6]

A multigravid woman, early in her second trimester, had been ill for 1 week with chest pain, yellow sputum, wheeze and breathlessness. She also had diarrhoea and vomiting. A locum GP called, heard crepitations and wheeze, diagnosed a chest infection and prescribed erythromycin and a linctus. The next day the patient was even more breathless, and another locum GP was called. He diagnosed acute bronchitis and prescribed salbutamol. Within 48 hours the patient was found dead by her husband. Autopsy showed widespread bronchopneumonia, and *Staphyloccocus aureus* was cultured from the pus.

LESSONS

- Appropriate education in the community is of vital importance.
- Pregnant women may be more susceptible to infection due to physiological changes. Healthcare workers in the community must be aware of this and be alert to the early signs of serious infections.
- The presence of diarrhoea and vomiting may often be a symptom of severe infection.
- A young pregnant woman who is not improving despite antibiotics should be referred to hospital without delay.

CASE 15 (2000–2002)[2]

This woman died of pneumonia. She attended her local Accident and Emergency department more than once with breathlessness and fever. She was eventually treated as if she had pulmonary embolism, for no good reason. The seriousness of her condition was not recognised until she was admitted to the maternity unit, delivered of a dead baby and found to be in severe cardiorespiratory failure.

LESSONS

- Breathlessness and fever are important signs of severe sepsis that were not recognised in this case. This patient required early resuscitation and early administration of antibiotics.

CASE 16 (2000–2002)[2]

In a case of mastitis, the junior doctors did not appreciate the gravity of the woman's condition. She was transferred to a hospital with a gynaecology unit but no maternity unit, without the knowledge of or consultation with senior staff. Advice from a consultant obstetrician was not sought until she was moribund in intensive care.

LESSONS

■ Appropriate advice from senior staff must be sought at an early stage.

Recommendations

Prevention

History has taught us that prevention of infection can be very effective. Basic hygiene, such as hand washing, and the use of alcohol-based rubs are vital. It is unclear whether topical vaginal antiseptics are of any benefit.[32,33] With regard to antibiotics, data from the Cochrane Library support the use of prophylactic antibiotics during Caesarean section.[25] The antibiotic used for prophylaxis should be limited to one dose, in order to reduce the possibility of resistance. When infection develops and the patient is systemically ill, urgent and repeated bacteriological specimens, including blood cultures, must be obtained. Parenteral antibiotics may need to be given before the diagnosis is confirmed. Antibiotics should be chosen on the basis of the likely source of infection, and guided by susceptibility patterns in the community and within the hospital. During pregnancy, antibiotics that are known to be safe for the fetus should be administered, such as the beta-lactams or aminoglycosides.

Communication

Communication is also vitally important. Junior staff must seek advice from senior staff at an early stage, and there must be timely involvement of the critical care services. The advice of a microbiologist must also be sought as soon as possible. Communication between the hospital and community teams is vital for identifying patients at particular risk of sepsis in both the antenatal and postnatal periods.

Education

One of the most frequent lessons to emerge from the case reports is the need for the education of staff in the early recognition of severe sepsis, and the need for the immediate institution of appropriate therapies to prevent progression to septic shock. It is interesting that in 1769, puerperal sepsis was common and all the signs and symptoms and the serious nature of the condition were well recognised.[4] It is rare today, but as the CEMD 1994–1996 report[7] states, it is not a disease of the past, and all staff both in hospital and in the community must once again be alert to the early clinical manifestations.

There is now training, such as the ALERT (Acute Life-threatening Events Recognition and Treatment) course, designed to educate staff in the recognition of critical illness. Such training focuses on the need for staff to identify organ impairment or failure as soon as possible, to initiate the simple treatment required to prevent the spiralling cascade to multi-organ failure, and to improve the communication skills necessary to facilitate further care.

Detection

In Accident and Emergency departments and on the wards there has recently been an emphasis on developing early warning scores[34,35] that help to identify critically ill patients and enable staff to alert the appropriate teams. A common mistake is to assume that a patient who is sitting up in bed talking cannot be critically ill. The clue is nearly always in the vital signs. Early warning scores allocate points to routine vital sign measurements on the basis of deviation from a normal range. Although there has not been a validated scoring system to account for the normal physiological values of pregnancy, the principle is the same as in the non-pregnant patient. The more abnormal the vital sign, the higher the score will be. If the score is above a certain level, the patient should be assessed by a doctor immediately. Clearly it is important to remember that heart rate increases early on in pregnancy to a maximum of 15–20 beats/min above baseline at term, and that the respiratory rate also becomes mildly elevated. Blood pressure decreases from early on, and reaches a nadir at about 16–24 weeks, from which time it increases slowly back to baseline levels. The hospital must have a clear policy that requires an appropriate clinical and communication response in the event of patient deterioration. The introduction of critical care outreach or medical emergency teams may help to improve outcomes,[36,37] as it will help to increase intensive-care involvement in patient management before admission to the ICU. It is also important to remember that doctors and midwives in the community require training to prevent sepsis, and to recognise it early when it does occur.

Guidelines for treatment

In 2003, critical care and infectious disease experts representing 11 international organisations developed management guidelines for severe sepsis and septic shock that would be of practical use for the bedside clinician, under the auspices of the 'Surviving Sepsis Campaign', an international effort to increase awareness and improve outcome in severe sepsis.[3] The guidelines are directed at a number of areas (*see also* Chapter 10, Box 10.2).

Resuscitation

The first recommendation is that resuscitation should begin as soon as the syndrome is recognised, and should not be delayed pending admission to the intensive-care unit. The goals identified for initial resuscitation using either crystalloids or colloids are listed in Box 9.1. It has been shown in a randomised, controlled, single-blinded study that resuscitation towards these goals in the initial 6 hours following presentation of patients to the Accident and Emergency department with septic shock reduces 28-day mortality.[38] It is not known whether this approach is applicable to the obstetric patient with septic shock, but the principles of treatment and monitoring are the same. It is necessary to exercise caution with fluid boluses, as these women may be more at risk of developing pulmonary oedema due to pregnancy-induced decreases in colloid osmotic pressure.[23]

> **BOX 9.1** The goals of initial resuscitation
> - Central venous pressure 8–12 mmHg.
> - Mean arterial pressure ≥ 65 mmHg.
> - Urine output ≥ 0.5 ml/kg/hour.
> - Central venous saturation (superior vena cava) or mixed venous oxygen saturation ≥ 70%.

Diagnosis

Appropriate cultures must be obtained before antibiotics are started. To optimise identification of the organisms, at least two blood cultures should be obtained. Cultures of other sites, including the placenta if necessary, should be obtained. Diagnostic studies may identify the source of infection.

Antibiotic therapy

Intravenous antibiotic therapy should be started within the first hour of recognition of severe sepsis, after appropriate cultures have been obtained. The antibiotics that are given should be based on hospital protocols and the likely nature of the infection. The regimen will need to be reassessed after 48–72 hours on the basis of microbiological and clinical data.

Source control

A patient who presents with severe sepsis should be evaluated for the presence of infection that is amenable to source control measures. Intervention should only be undertaken following adequate resuscitation. Timely intervention is of particular importance in patients with necrotising soft tissue infection or intestinal ischaemia.

Fluid therapy

Fluid resuscitation may consist of either crystalloids or colloids. There is no evidence base for one type of fluid over another. Fluid resuscitation may be given to those with hypovolaemia at a rate of 500–1,000 ml of crystalloid or 300–500 ml of colloid over 30 minutes, and repeated depending on the response. As stated above, particular care must be taken when fluid resuscitating the obstetric patient.

Vasopressors

Vasopressors may be required to reverse hypotension if the fluid challenge fails to restore adequate perfusion pressure rapidly.

Further recommendations relate mainly to the care in an intensive-care environment, and will not be documented here. They include recommendations for the use of steroids, recombinant human activated protein C and blood product administration. There are also recommendations for ventilation, sedation, glucose control, renal replacement, bicarbonate therapy, deep vein thrombosis prophylaxis and stress ulcer prophylaxis. Once again these recommendations may not all be applicable to the obstetric patient – particularly, for example, the patient who may still be pregnant with a live fetus. The use of steroids in these patients may increase the risk of further infection.

Conclusion

Sepsis remains an important cause of death in the obstetric population. Until recently there has been a lack of standard care for these patients. However, the introduction of courses that enable recognition of septic patients, together with the introduction of guidelines directed at early management, will hopefully decrease mortality in the ensuing years.

CHAPTER 10

Intensive care

TOM CLUTTON-BROCK

A chapter dedicated to intensive-care issues in maternal deaths first appeared in the 1991–1993 triennial CEMD report,[1] and has been a regular feature in subsequent reports. For each of the periods for which data are available, approximately 30% of all maternal deaths involved admission to an intensive-care unit. Deaths directly attributable to poor intensive care appear to be rare. However, cases where a delay in referral or admission to intensive care may have contributed to a maternal death are more commonly cited.

This chapter looks not only at lessons to be learned from maternal deaths in intensive care, but also at the broader picture of the role of intensive care in the management of the sick mother. In particular, it explores the role that a better understanding of the management of severely disturbed physiology can have in reducing maternal mortality.

The origins of the principles of intensive care can be traced back to Florence Nightingale, who proposed the collection of the sickest patients into one area in order to improve staff:patient ratios. These principles were applied to the management of casualties during both world wars, and the introduction of positive pressure ventilation followed the poliomyelitis epidemic in Copenhagen in 1952.

The last 50 or so years have seen intensive care grow steadily from the province of a small number of enthusiasts to a major specialty in its own right. Comprehensive training programmes have been introduced, and the recommendations that units should be managed by consultants with dedicated intensive-care sessions have been widely implemented. A useful introduction has been the categorisation of intensive-care beds into three levels, based on patient dependency, as shown in Box 10.1.[2]

The provision of intensive-care beds increased steadily over the 6 years between 1999 and 2005, stimulated in part by the comprehensive review undertaken by the Department of Health in 1999 and published in 2000.[3] The report by the Critical Care Stakeholder Forum, entitled *Quality Critical Care,*[4] cites a figure of 3,193 open intensive-care beds in England for July 2005, an increase of 35% since July 2000. The majority of this increase was represented by the provision of level 2 (HDU) beds. A reply by the Secretary of State for Health to the House of Commons in May 2005

BOX 10.1 Levels of critical care

Level 0
Patients whose needs can be met through normal ward care in an acute hospital.

Level 1
Patients at risk of their condition deteriorating, or those recently relocated from higher levels of care whose needs can be met on an acute ward with additional advice and support from the critical care team.

Level 2
Patients requiring more detailed observation or intervention, including support for a single failing organ system or postoperative care, and those stepping down from higher levels of care.

Level 3
Patients needing monitoring and support for two or more organ systems, one of which may be basic or advanced respiratory support.

Adapted from www.ics.ac.uk/downloads/icsstandards-levelsofca.pdf

---

stated that the number of open NHS adult intensive-care (level 1) beds in January 2005 was 1,787.[5]

Despite these encouraging figures, the pressures on intensive-care beds continue, there has been little reduction in the number of transfers to a unit outside the referring hospital, and the number of operations cancelled due to lack of availability of an intensive-care bed has, if anything, risen slightly.[4] This all translates into high bed occupancies, and reduces the availability of beds for emergency admissions from obstetric units.

The high cost of intensive care means that occupancy rates are unlikely to fall. Thus reduced bed availability and delays in admission should be expected by all involved in the referral of emergency admissions. Some of these issues have been addressed by the introduction of outreach teams, and *Quality Critical Care*[4] recommends that these should be expanded to provide 24-hour cover, 7 days a week.

Outcomes from intensive care in obstetrics

Until recently, the largest obstetric data set from the UK was that reported by Hazelgrove *et al.*,[6] who reported an analysis of the South West Thames database, which collects data on admissions to 14 general critical care units. They identified 1.8% of all admissions (210 out of 11,385 cases) as related to pregnancy. In 2005, the Intensive Care National Audit and Research Centre (ICNARC) published a study looking at the case mix, outcome and activity of obstetric admissions to adult general critical care units.[7]

Of 219,468 admissions in the ICNARC Case Mix Programme Database (CMPD), 1452 (0.7%) were identified as direct obstetric admissions and 450 were indirect or coincidental obstetric admissions (0.2% of all CMPD admissions). A comparative group of non-obstetric female admissions aged 16–50 years consisted of 22,938 admissions (10.5% of all CMPD admissions). In total, the 1902 obstetric admissions represented 0.9% of all CMPD admissions and 7.7% of all female admissions aged 16–50 years. The trend in obstetric admissions over time (as a percentage of all admissions) for the 7 complete years from 1996 to 2002 inclusive shows no significant trend over time, even after adjusting for the changing units participating in the CMP (odds ratio = 0.96 per year, 95% confidence interval (CI) = 0.94–1.01). Thus, on average, 9 in 1,000 intensive-care admissions will be young and potentially fit obstetric patients, and a large unit will admit 5 to 6 patients each year. However, in relation to other conditions, intensive-care specialists will have minimal exposure to critically ill obstetric patients.

Similarly, only a very small proportion of obstetric patients will require intensive care. Bouvier-Colle et al.[8] studied 435 obstetric patients admitted to intensive care and calculated that the frequency was 36 per 100,000 live births. Of these, mortality was lower for scheduled maternity cases. In a Canadian study conducted by Baskett and Sternadel[9] over 14 years between 1980 and 1993, a total of 76,119 women were delivered, with two maternal deaths (2.6 per 100,000). In total, 55 women required transfer for critical care (0.7 per 1,000). The main reasons for transfer were hypertensive disease (25%), haemorrhage (22%) and sepsis (15%). Wheatley et al.[10] reviewed the predictability of admissions to their ICU, and found that 67% of patients had no previous medical or obstetric history. As in other series, the major reasons for admission were hypertensive disorders of pregnancy (66%) and haemorrhage (19%), with 79% of cases following Caesarean section and 40% requiring ventilatory support. On the basis of these figures, it is estimated that a busy obstetric unit with say 6,500 deliveries per year will on average send 5 patients to intensive care each year.

Another important finding from the ICNARC review of obstetric patients in intensive care was the low mortality observed in obstetric patients. The South West Thames study had reported a mortality of 3.3%. The ICNARC study found that 2.2% of patients who were direct obstetric admissions died before ultimate discharge from hospital, compared with 6.0% of indirect or coincidental obstetric admissions and 19.6% of female non-obstetric admissions aged 16–50 years (χ^2 test, $P < 0.001$). In other words, over 96% of obstetric admissions to intensive care survive.

It is of course possible that the obstetric patients are overall a fitter group than the age-matched control group. The ICNARC study showed that the widely used Acute Physiology and Chronic Health Evaluation (APACHE) II severity scoring and mortality prediction model was poorly calibrated for obstetric patients, and significantly overestimated their risk of death. This would support the view that this group of patients has a better outcome than is predicted by any existing model.

Thus consideration of the methods and timing of referral is more likely to produce useful lessons for those caring for the sick mother than just observing the small numbers who die in intensive care. Some have questioned the value of maternal morbidity studies in the developed world. For example, Waterstone *et al.*[11] measured severe morbidity as opposed to mortality in 19 maternity units within the South East Thames region and six neighbouring hospitals caring for pregnant women from the region between 1 March 1997 and 28 February 1998. A total of 48,865 women were studied during this time period. The authors reported 588 cases of severe obstetric morbidity, giving an incidence of 12 in 1,000 deliveries. In contrast, there were only five maternal deaths attributed to the conditions studied. Disease-specific morbidities per 1,000 deliveries were 6.7 for severe haemorrhage, 3.9 for severe pre-eclampsia, 0.2 for eclampsia, 0.5 for HELLP (haemolysis, elevated liver enzymes, low platelets) syndrome, 0.4 for severe sepsis and 0.2 for uterine rupture. Age over 34 years, non-white ethnic group, past or current hypertension, previous postpartum haemorrhage, delivery by emergency Caesarean section, antenatal admission to hospital, multiple pregnancy, social exclusion, and taking iron or antidepressants at antenatal booking were all independently associated with morbidity after adjustment. Most of these factors are also associated with excess maternal mortality.

Facilitating intensive care

A common theme in CEMD reports is delay either in referring patients to intensive care or in achieving admission. There are important lessons to be learned from both anticipated and unexpected admissions.

Planned admissions to intensive care

We have already seen[10] that over two-thirds of obstetric patients admitted to intensive care have no previous medical or obstetric history. However, there are patients for whom a significant risk of post-delivery complications can be anticipated and admission to intensive care can be reasonably predicted. The rarity of obstetric admissions to intensive care means that this process requires careful planning by all involved.

Early multi-disciplinary meetings are essential, and should involve consultant obstetricians, consultant anaesthetists, consultant intensive-care specialists, senior midwives and senior intensive-care nurses, as well as consultants from any other specialties involved (e.g. cardiology, renal medicine, rheumatology, etc.) and other professional groups as appropriate. The mother, of course, is also a key component in the planning, and discussions of risk and the development of appropriate plans should be undertaken at regular intervals as pregnancy proceeds. It may be most appropriate to identify key individuals to undertake these discussions in a clear and compassionate fashion.

Severe cardiac disease is a good model of the need for this approach. Previous CEMD reports have been critical of cases in which there was little or no attempt to make appropriate plans for multi-disciplinary care.[12]

In Case 2 in Chapter 7 of this book, the management of the patient's pregnancy is criticised, but in particular it is stated that:

Patients with pulmonary vascular disease have a high risk of dying, particularly after delivery. A multi-disciplinary team should plan their management. However, no anaesthetist was consulted about her until she arrived on the labour ward. No invasive monitoring was used.

It seems reasonable to assume that there was no intensive-care involvement in the planning of this patient's care.

Smith et al.[13] describe the outcomes and costs of five cases of severe cardiac disease in pregnancy. One of these patients was a young mother with a history of severe pulmonary hypertension following multiple pulmonary emboli against a background of systemic lupus erythematosus. Her care was planned with input from the obstetricians, anaesthetists, cardiologist, rheumatologist, intensive-care specialist, midwives and intensive-care nurses. A decision was made to continue with intravenous anticoagulation because of the high risks of further pulmonary embolus, and to deliver the baby electively at 37 weeks by Caesarean section under general anaesthesia. Pre-operative trans-thoracic echocardiography showed a severely dilated right ventricle and estimated pulmonary artery pressures at systemic levels. A date and time for the section were arranged in advance and an intensive-care bed was booked. This all sounds very straightforward, but the Critical Care Stakeholder Forum report[4] cited earlier reports a 12% incidence of cancellation of urgent surgery due to a lack of intensive-care beds, and this needs to be considered when booking obstetric cases into intensive care in advance of a procedure.

It is of course entirely possible that the intensive-care specialist primarily involved in the multi-disciplinary team planning is not the one in charge of the unit on or immediately before the planned day of admission. Therefore careful communication is required if the process is to run smoothly. In the above case, an ICU bed was kept for the patient and operative care was managed by a consultant obstetrician, two consultant and two trainee obstetric anaesthetists, and a consultant intensive-care specialist with experience of anaesthesia for cardiac surgery. Invasive monitoring, including pulmonary artery catheterisation with semi-continuous cardiac output monitoring and continuous mixed venous saturation monitoring, was instituted prior to induction of anaesthesia. Nitric oxide by inhalation and intravenous prostacyclin were used as prophylaxis against any further rise in pulmonary vascular resistance. (The role of pulmonary artery catheterisation in the care of sick mothers is discussed later.) The Caesarean section proceeded uneventfully and the patient was transferred by ambulance 600 yards to the intensive-care unit across the road. Unfortunately, she returned to the operating theatre 2 days later for evacuation of a wound haematoma, and suffered a cardiac arrest at induction. Extensive resuscitation attempts were unsuccessful in restoring a cardiac output, demonstrating the dangerous nature of this disease.

Emergency admissions to intensive care

Emergencies will represent the majority of admissions. Typical scenarios are unexpectedly heavy bleeding during or after a Caesarean section, requiring significant transfusion of red cells and blood products, or severe pre-eclampsia with reduced urine output, evidence of pulmonary oedema and challenging blood pressure control. If an ICU bed is not immediately available, it is important that discussions take place at a senior level as soon as possible, and if a delay is inevitable, a detailed plan of care during the waiting period should be discussed.

In the latest CEMD report,[14] evidence was cited from case reports that on occasion the care of the sick mother between the time when the need for intensive care was identified and actual arrival on the ICU was sub-optimal. In particular, some patients who went on to die arrived with significant clotting disturbances and evidence of only small volumes of clotting products having been transfused. In other cases, patients had deteriorated significantly while waiting, and required urgent intubation on arrival. Clearly some of these situations are unavoidable, while others would have benefited from a better dialogue between obstetric anaesthetic staff and the intensive-care staff (in both directions). It is important to understand that intensive care should be part of a continuum of care and not a stepwise change in the nature of the care provided. To illustrate this, it is useful to review what a modern intensive-care unit has to offer the sick mother, and how the processes that are used can be started before admission.

Nursing ratios

The current levels of intensive-care dependency are shown in Box 10.1. Level 3 patients are typically nursed at staff:patient ratios of 1:1, and level 2 patients at ratios of 1:2, with trained intensive-care nursing staff for both levels. It is important not to underestimate the enormous difference between this level of nursing care and that typically provided on an open obstetric ward. Indeed it is this level of nursing dependency and expertise which is at the heart of intensive care. Intensive-care staff are often critical of the care provided for patients on a standard ward, but this often fails to take into account the enormous advantages provided by 1:1 nursing. There is another equally important point to be made, namely that a small ward or even a cubicle that has been equipped with monitoring equipment and perhaps a ventilator does not represent an intensive-care unit. Monitoring, sophisticated ventilators, etc. make intensive care easier, but it is the experience and the intensity of the nursing care provided that make intensive care what it is. Delivery units typically provide highly experienced 1:1 care, so there is the potential to deliver similar care if appropriate training and support were provided.

Monitoring
Arterial pressure

In some respects much of intensive care is about control – the control required to return severely disturbed physiology to within acceptable parameters and then to maintain control while the body undergoes complex and often only partially understood repair.

Blood pressure control, blood gas control and fluid balance are good examples of this. Around 12 million arterial cannulas are inserted into patients worldwide each year. They dramatically improve the control of blood pressure in the sick patient, and provide access for regular blood gas and other samples. Most anaesthetists in training will have had considerable experience in their insertion, and with appropriate care the benefits of their use far outweigh the risks. Adverse events are primarily caused by the inadvertent injection of drugs into the cannula. However, the use of dedicated and coloured sets should help to reduce this problem. Cannulas are easier to insert before profound hypotension sets in. If there is more than a minimal risk of significant blood loss, and in anything other than mild pre-eclampsia, arterial pressure monitoring should be started early on. The finding that oscillometric measurements of blood pressure may give inaccurate diastolic readings in pre-eclampsia is not a new one.[15] The recently published *Report of the Independent Advisory Group on Blood Pressure Monitoring in Clinical Practice*[16] contains the following recommendation:

> In those clinical conditions where oscillometry is inappropriate (e.g. arrhythmias, pre-eclampsia and certain vascular diseases), an alternative method of pressure measurement (auscultation, arterial cannulation) should be used.

Central venous pressure (CVP)

CVP monitoring is almost universal in intensive care and in anaesthesia for major surgery. The indications for CVP monitoring are the requirement to measure filling pressures in the right side of the circulation as an indication of the adequacy of circulating blood volume, and for the administration of vasoconstricting inotropes or hyperosmolar or hyperoncotic fluids. The internal jugular and subclavian routes have the highest success rate for placing a cannula in the superior vena cava, but the subclavian route carries a slightly higher risk of pneumothorax. Both routes involve finding a vein that lies next to an artery, so both carry a risk of arterial puncture. In 2002, the National Institute for Clinical Excellence (NICE)[17] issued guidance that, where possible, central venous access should be obtained using ultrasound guidance. The equipment for this is widely available, and obstetric units which regularly insert CVP lines should consider purchasing the equipment and providing suitable training. Carotid puncture during attempted internal jugular cannulation is not uncommon. Once recognised, unless there is a severe coagulopathy, it should be reasonably easy to manage. The CEMD 1991–1993 report[18] records a case in which attempted internal jugular cannulation caused a haematoma, leading to fatal tracheal compression (*see* Case 15 in Chapter 6). In the presence of a coagulopathy or severe thrombocytopenia, puncture of the subclavian artery can lead to life-threatening intra-thoracic haemorrhage.

CVP monitoring is not a treatment but a monitoring tool which, although useful in the management of fluid replacement in severe haemorrhage, should not delay the appropriate treatment. CVP will of course often be low in the presence of severe haemorrhage, making the detection of the veins in the neck even more challenging. Unless peripheral venous access is impossible, CVP lines are not suitable for the rapid transfusion of red cells or blood products. Although modern quad-lumen lines have a 14-gauge lumen, they are much longer than peripheral cannulas, therefore increasing the resistance to flow. In addition, red cell concentrates are stored at 4°C and may have an elevated potassium concentration. Their rapid transfusion under pressure directly through the right atrium into the right ventricle can produce asystole.

The interpretation of CVP readings is also not always straightforward. A low CVP indicates inadequate circulating blood volume or vasodilatation (or both). In contrast, a 'normal' or slightly elevated CVP does not always indicate adequate circulating volume. The vasoconstriction that accompanies blood loss will artificially elevate the CVP, as will the use of inotropes and vasoconstrictors. Particularly after a significant bleed the CVP should be interpreted with caution, and other measures of the adequacy of circulating blood volume, such as urine output, peripheral warming and correction of acid–base balance, should be used.

Pulmonary artery catheters

In practice, the indications for pulmonary artery catheterisation are straightforward, and can be summarised as follows:

- patients in whom a difference between right- and left-sided filling pressures is expected
- for the measurement of cardiac output
- for the measurement of mixed venous oxygen saturation.

Despite this, the use of this monitoring tool varies enormously between intensive-care units, even when the different case mix of patients is taken into account. A recent survey by ICNARC, quoted in an editorial by Young,[19] showed rates ranging from 3% to 76% of admissions in a recent survey of 69 ICUs in the UK. In 1996, a paper by Connors *et al.*[20] appeared to demonstrate that pulmonary artery catheterisation might actually increase mortality and morbidity in intensive-care patients. The result was a heated debate but few if any definitive answers. ICNARC managed a UK-based randomised trial designed to assess the clinical effectiveness of pulmonary artery catheters in the management of patients in intensive care (PAC-Man). Just over 1,000 ICU patients were randomised to receive a pulmonary artery catheter or not, and the effect on outcome was studied. The results, which were published in 2005,[21] reached the following conclusion:

> Our findings indicate no clear evidence of benefit or harm by managing critically ill patients with a PAC. Efficacy studies are needed to ascertain whether management protocols involving PAC use can result in improved outcomes in specific groups, if these devices are not to become a redundant technology.

The number of obstetric patients in this study will have been very small, but it illustrates an important principle, namely that monitoring alone is not associated with an improvement in outcome.

Cardiac output

The measurement of cardiac output is another procedure that is usually confined to the intensive-care unit, thermodilution using a pulmonary artery catheter still being considered by most to be the current gold standard. More recently, other dye dilution techniques using either cold injectates and arterial thermistors or lithium ion-selective electrodes have been introduced into clinical practice. Trans-oesophageal Doppler measurements have also enjoyed an increase in popularity. All of these techniques still remain better suited to the intensive-care environment. There are two new techniques for estimating cardiac output which have a much wider applicability. Both of them are based on modifications of much older methods.

Pulse contour estimation of stroke volume (and, when multiplied by the heart rate, the cardiac output) from the arterial pressure waveform was originally described many years ago. It has been available as pulse contour cardiac output (PCCO) as part of dye dilution systems, but has until recently required calibration against invasive measurements of cardiac output on a regular basis. The Vigileo monitor (marketed by Edwards Lifesciences, Irvine, CA, USA) uses a dedicated arterial pressure transducer which, in addition to providing a conventional arterial waveform, analyses the waveform to derive stroke volume. The basis for the algorithm is the physiological premise that pulse pressure is proportional to stroke volume. It is also known that aortic compliance, a significant determinant of vascular tone, is inversely proportional to pulse pressure for a given stroke volume. The system uses an internal database consisting of a very large number of known stroke volumes and pulse pressures obtained from ICU patients, which removes the need for invasive calibration. In practice all that is required is an arterial cannula, so the method would be very applicable in obstetric theatres. Care should be exercised until the accuracy and precision of this device in widespread practice have been established.

An even less invasive method involves the re-launch of impedance cardiography monitoring (ICG). This technique involves placing two pairs of ECG electrodes on the neck and lower thorax. In the past ICG has suffered from unacceptably poor precision of measurement, but advances in hardware and software with the latest-generation ICG monitor (BioZ; CardioDynamics, San Diego, CA, USA), including digital signal processing (DISQ digital impedance signal quantifier; CardioDynamics, San Diego, CA, USA) and the creation of a proprietary modification to the Sramek–Bernstein equation (ZMARC impedance-modulating aortic compliance) have yielded significantly better results.[22] However, further evidence is needed to confirm the levels of accuracy and precision required in clinical practice.

Pregnancy adds an extra complication to the interpretation of cardiac output measurements, and we may have to revisit these if cardiac output monitoring is to be more widely used as less invasive systems appear. Cardiac output increases early in pregnancy (e.g. by 13–20% by 5–11 weeks' gestation). The early changes are attributed to an increase in stroke volume, and are independent of metabolic rate and pregnancy-induced increases in blood volume. The early increase in cardiac output may be triggered by a decrease in systemic vascular resistance (SVR). Cardiac output continues to increase throughout pregnancy. Peak values (27–50% higher than baseline) occur late in the second trimester.

During the third trimester, the change in cardiac output is highly variable. Pooled data indicate a decrease, but data for individual women indicate an increase, a decrease, or no change.[23] This variability may reflect changes related to body position (e.g. a decrease in stroke volume due to compression of the inferior vena cava when the pregnant woman is supine) or to the technique used to measure the output.

Cardiac output should be measured with the pregnant woman in the same position (e.g. left lateral decubitus, *not* supine), because output is lower in supine and standing positions. The use of cardiac index is equivocal, because the correlation between cardiac output and body surface area during pregnancy is poor.

Mixed and central venous oxygen saturation

Mixed venous oxygen saturation measured from blood in the pulmonary artery has been widely used in ICUs for many years, and systems are available for making continuous measurements through a pulmonary artery catheter. The saturation represents the balance between oxygen delivery (determined primarily from haemoglobin concentration, cardiac output and arterial saturation) and oxygen uptake. All of these are altered in pregnancy, but in general the balance between delivery and consumption is preserved in the healthy patient. Of interest has been the recent rediscovery that there exists a useful relationship between central venous and mixed venous saturation, and that central venous saturation measurements may be useful for directing the management of certain groups of patients.[24,25] As a result of these publications there has been a notable increase in the use of central venous saturation measurements in many ICU patients. These measurements might be useful in obstetric patients who have a central line in place.

Surviving Sepsis Campaign

The Institute for Healthcare Improvement in the USA states:

> Mortality associated with severe sepsis remains unacceptably high: 30 to 50 per cent. When shock is present, mortality is reported to be even higher: 50 to 60 per cent. There are approximately 750,000 new sepsis cases each year, with at least 210,000 fatalities. As medicine becomes more aggressive, with invasive procedures and immunosuppression, the incidence of sepsis is likely to increase even more. The Surviving Sepsis Campaign – a partnership of the Society of Critical Care Medicine, the European Society of Intensive Care Medicine, and the International Sepsis Forum – has teamed up with the Institute for Healthcare Improvement to wage war on sepsis and achieve a 25 per cent reduction in sepsis mortality within five years (by 2009).[26]

This is of relevance to obstetrics, as sepsis is an important cause of critical illness in this group of patients, and CEMD reports include a chapter devoted to death from sepsis. The campaign is based on delivering a standardised bundle of care. Although much of this care will be delivered in the intensive-care unit, the resuscitation component should be started as soon as possible, and this may well be on an obstetric ward or in an obstetric theatre. The details of the resuscitation bundle are listed in Box 10.2, and discussed in Chapter 9 of this book.

Outreach

Following the publication of *Comprehensive Critical Care* in 2000,[3] there has been a rapid increase in the provision of intensive-care outreach services. Here senior members of the intensive-care nursing staff, usually with senior intensive-care medical cover, provide a service to the normal wards. This service may include a component of acute pain management, but is designed to review any patient who is sufficiently unwell to warrant additional input, and the process often allows for earlier referral to the intensive-care unit proper. The service has been well received, and should be considered in the context of obstetrics. Clearly the low rate of admissions would suggest that outreach services may be limited, but late referrals have featured in recent CEMD reports.

Early Warning Scoring (EWS) systems

Complaints about delayed referral to intensive care and delays in recognising the sick patient are certainly not confined to obstetrics. This has led to the introduction of a number of Early Warning Scoring (EWS) systems, also known as Patient at Risk Scores (PARS) or Modified Early Warning Scores (MEWS).[26] An EWS is calculated for a patient using five simple physiological variables, namely mental response, pulse

---

BOX 10.2 Sepsis resuscitation bundle[26]

(A 'bundle' is a group of interventions related to a disease process that, when executed together, result in better outcomes than when they are implemented individually.)

- Serum lactate measured.
- Blood cultures obtained prior to antibiotic administration.
- From the time of presentation, broad-spectrum antibiotics administered within 3 hours for Accident and Emergency admissions and 1 hour for non-Accident and Emergency ICU admissions.
- In the event of hypotension and/or lactate > 4 mmol/l (36 mg/dl):
  - deliver an initial minimum of 20 ml/kg of crystalloid (or colloid equivalent)
  - apply vasopressors for hypotension that is not responding to initial fluid resuscitation, to maintain mean arterial pressure (MAP) > 65 mmHg.
- In the event of persistent hypotension despite fluid resuscitation (septic shock) and/or lactate > 4 mmol/l (36 mg/dl):
  - achieve central venous pressure (CVP) of > 8 mmHg
  - achieve central venous oxygen saturation ($S_{cv}O_2$) of > 70%.

rate, systolic blood pressure, respiratory rate and temperature. For patients who are postoperative or unwell enough to be catheterised, a sixth variable, namely urine output, can be added. The principle is that small changes in these five variables combined will be seen earlier using EWS than by waiting for obvious changes in individual variables – such as a marked drop in systolic blood pressure, which is often a pre-terminal event. Of all the variables, respiratory rate is the most important for assessing the clinical state of a patient, but it is the one that is least often recorded. Respiratory rate is thought to be the most sensitive indicator of a patient's physio- logical well-being. A typical EWS scoring system is shown in Table 10.1. The changes in physiology that are seen in normal pregnancy mean that any scoring system may need to be modified for this group of patients. The poor calibration of scoring systems for obstetric admissions supports this theory,[7] but does mean that the error will be on the safe side (i.e. mothers will be referred earlier than may be necessary).

TABLE 10.1   Example of early warning scoring (EWS) system[26]

SCORE	3	2	1	0	1	2	3
Heart rate (beats/min)		< 40	41–50	51–100	101–110	111–129	
Systolic blood pressure (mmHg)	< 70	71–80	81–100	101–199		> 200	
Respiration rate (breaths/min)		< 8		9–14	15–20	21–29	>30
CNS				Alert	Drowsy/ rousable to voice or newly confused	Responds to pain	Unresponsive
Temperature (°C)		< 35		35.1–37.5	> 37.5		
Urine	Nil	< 20 ml/2 hours	20–50 ml/2 hours or has not voided within 4 hours of admission	> 50 ml/2 hours			

Quality of intensive care provided

There is evidence of difficulties with regard to the care that is provided in intensive care after a sick mother has been admitted.

CASE 1 (1997–1999)[12]

This patient, of high parity and a smoker, bled at delivery. There was difficulty with transfusion because of antibodies, and she had a significant postpartum haemorrhage (PPH). During examination under anaesthesia, she developed bronchospasm and pulmonary oedema. Fluid overload was suspected, as a large volume of Gelofusine® (Braun) had been given. The patient was transferred to the ICU, where she developed a coagulopathy. Although bronchospasm improved, oxygenation remained a problem. Chest X-ray showed pulmonary oedema, so frusemide was given and ventilatory support was escalated. She became stable over the next few days, but a few days after delivery she became oliguric, despite cardiovascular stability. She was transferred to a regional centre for renal support. Tracheostomy was performed to expedite weaning off the ventilator, but problems of bleeding from the tracheostomy site developed, although the patient continued to wean from ventilation. A few days later she became acutely hypoxic and a suction catheter could not be passed through the tracheostomy tube. Fibre-optic bronchoscopy suggested a suboptimal position of the tracheostomy. Ventilatory support was reintroduced, formal revision of the tracheostomy was suggested, and the patient was returned to theatre next day for this purpose. A size 8 endotracheal tube was passed, but did not bypass the tracheostomy stoma sufficiently to ventilate the patient. A smaller tube was passed, but did not result in satisfactory ventilation, so a size 8 tube was again attempted, but there was no chest movement, nor was there CO_2 elimination. Hypoxia and hypotension required adrenaline. All attempts to obtain access to the trachea failed. Tracheobronchial fistula was suspected, and the cardiothoracic surgeons were contacted, but despite all attempts to provide a secure airway, the patient remained severely hypoxic and died. At autopsy, the soft tissues around the tracheostomy site were haemorrhagic, with a 1-cm tear in the right main bronchus and copious blood in the airways, in addition to changes of ARDS.

This story is tragic, as it appears that the patient was recovering from other organ system failures and might have been expected to recover. This case was also discussed in the haemorrhage chapter of the same report, where her intensive care was described as 'excellent.'

Delays in admission and poor record keeping are also found in cases reported by the CEMD.

CASE 2 (1997–1999)[12]

This patient, who spoke no English, sustained a massive PPH from multiple vaginal tears, and subsequently developed a vescicovaginal fistula after a hysterectomy, which was repaired many months later. After this operation she was over-transfused and developed dilutional hyponatraemia as a result of receiving 5 litres of dextrose/saline overnight (to force a diuresis in the presence of oliguria). She had a fit on the ward, followed by a cardiorespiratory arrest, and was intubated and ventilated. No intensive-care bed was available on site, so she was transferred to another hospital for intensive care, and died a few days later without recovering consciousness. Prior to her collapse her plasma sodium level was 122 mmol/litre and her potassium level was 2.5 mmol/litre.

The author of this chapter in the CEMD report indicates that there were no records of the intensive-care management of this patient, making it difficult to assess the quality of the care that was provided. The latest CEMD report also found instances of poor or missing intensive-care records, although the standard of overall record keeping was good.

Conclusions

The need to admit a mother to intensive care is a rare event, and those that are admitted have a better than expected chance of survival. Successive CEMD reports have highlighted delays in admission, poor planning and sub-optimal care while waiting for an ICU bed. However, the processes of critical care can be initiated before admission to intensive care, and all anaesthetists caring for obstetric patients should be competent in the fundamentals of resuscitation and the restoration of disordered physiology. Early advice from intensive-care colleagues is useful. Modern intensive care is a sophisticated and sometimes complex specialty, but much of it is based on basic principles delivered with great attention to detail and requiring high staff to patient ratios.

New forms of cardiovascular monitoring may find a role in the detection and subsequent care of these patients, as may the use of modified early warning systems. Outreach has taken intensive care out of its physical box and delivered obvious benefit to many clinical areas. Its role in obstetrics should be explored by all units that admit potentially sick mothers.

References

CHAPTER 1 Saving mothers' lives

1 Callagan W. Epilogue. In: *Strategies to Reduce Pregnancy-Related Deaths. From identification and review to action.* Washington, DC: Centers for Disease Control and Prevention, American College of Obstetricians and Gynecologists; 2001.

2 Department of Health. *Why Mothers Die. Report on the Confidential Enquiries into Maternal Deaths in the United Kingdom, 1994–96.* London: The Stationery Office; 1998.

3 Pattinson R, editor. *Saving Mothers. The Second Report of the Confidential Enquiries into Maternal Deaths in South Africa, 1991–2001.* Pretoria: Department of Health; 2002.

4 Ministry of Health. *Report of the Confidential Enquiry into Maternal Deaths in England and Wales, 1952–1954. Reports on Public Health and Medical Subjects No.97.* London: HMSO; 1954.

5 Department of Health. *The Confidential Enquiries into Maternal and Child Health. Why Mothers Die, 2000–2002. The Sixth Report on the Confidential Enquiries into Maternal Deaths in the United Kingdom.* London: RCOG Press; 2004; www.cemach.org.uk

6 Department of Health for England. *The National Service Framework for Children, Young People and Maternity Services.* London: Department of Health; 2004.

7 United Nations. *Millennium Declaration.* New York: United Nations; 2000; www.un.org/millennium/declaration

8 World Health Organization. *Make Every Mother and Child Count. Annual Report 2005.* Geneva: World Health Organization; 2005.

9 World Health Organization. *Beyond the Numbers: reviewing maternal deaths and complications to make pregnancy safer.* Geneva: World Health Organization; 2004; www.who.int/reproductive-health

10 Lewis G. Pregnancy: reducing maternal death and disability. *Br Med Bull.* 2003; **67**: 27–37.

11 Kinloch JP, Smith J, Steven JA. *Maternal Mortality. Report on maternal mortality in Aberdeen, 1927–28, with special reference to puerperal sepsis.* Edinburgh: Scottish Board of Health; 1928.

12 Godber G. The Confidential Enquiry into Maternal Deaths. In: *A Question of Quality?* London: Nuffield Provincial Hospitals Trusts, and Oxford: Oxford University Press; 1976.

13 McFarlane A. Enquiries into maternal deaths in the twentieth century. In: *Why Mothers Die, 1997–99. The Fifth Report on the Confidential Enquiries into Maternal Deaths in the United Kingdom.* London: RCOG Press; 2001.

14 Ruststein D, Berenberg W, Chalmers T *et al.* Measuring the quality of care: a clinical method. *NEJM.* 1976; **294**: 582–8.

15 Department of Health and Social Security. *Report on Confidential Enquiries into Maternal Deaths in England and Wales, 1982–84. Reports on Health and Social Subjects No. 34.* London: HMSO; 1989.

16 Ministry of Health. *Report on Confidential Enquiries into Maternal Deaths in England and Wales, 1955–57. Reports on Public Health and Medical Subjects No. 103.* London: HMSO; 1960.

17 Ministry of Health. *Report on Confidential Enquiries into Maternal Deaths in England and Wales, 1958–60. Reports on Public Health and Medical Subjects No. 108.* London: HMSO; 1963.

18 Royal College of Obstetricians and Gynaecologists. *Report of the RCOG Working Party on Prophylaxis Against Thromboembolism in Gynaecology and Obstetrics.* London: RCOG Press; 1995.

19 Royal College of Obstetricians and Gynaecologists. *Thromboprophylaxis During Pregnancy, Labour and After Normal Vaginal Delivery. Guideline No. 37.* London: RCOG Press; 2004.

20 Department of Health. *Responding to Domestic Abuse: a handbook for health professionals.* London: Central Office of Information; 2006.

CHAPTER 2 General anaesthesia and failure to ventilate

1 Garcia-Rio F, Pino JM, Gomez L *et al.* Regulation of breathing and perception of dyspnea in healthy pregnant women. *Chest.* 1996; **100**: 446–53.

2 Pernoll ML, Metcalfe J, Schlenker TL *et al.* Oxygen consumption at rest and during exercise in pregnancy. *Respir Physiol.* 1975; **25**: 285–93.

3 Henderson JJ, Popat MT, Latto IP *et al.* Difficult Airway Society guidelines for management of the unanticipated difficult intubation. *Anaesthesia.* 2004; **59**: 675–94.

4 Klein JG. Five pitfalls in decisions about diagnosis and prescribing. *BMJ.* 2005; **330**: 781–3.

5 Bell D. Avoiding adverse outcomes when faced with 'difficulty with ventilation'. *Anaesthesia.* 2003; **58**: 945–8.

6 Webster CS. The nuclear power industry as an alternative analogy for safety in anaesthesia and a novel approach for the conceptualisation of safety goals. *Anaesthesia.* 2005; **60**: 1115–22.

7 Chiron B, Laffon M, Ferrandiere M *et al.* Standard preoxygenation technique versus two rapid techniques in pregnant patients. *Int J Obstet Anesthesia.* 2004; **13**: 11–14.

8 Hart EM, Owen H. Errors and omissions in anesthesia: a pilot study using a pilot's checklist. *Anesth Analg.* 2005; **101**: 246–50.

9 American Heart Association. Pediatric advanced life support. *Circulation.* 2005; **112**: 167–87.

10 Vanner RG, Asai T. Safe use of cricoid pressure. *Anaesthesia.* 1999; **54**: 1–3.

11 Yamamoto K, Tsubokawa T, Ohmura S *et al.* Left-molar approach improves the laryngeal view in patients with difficult laryngoscopy. *Anesthesiology.* 2000; **92**: 70–4.

12 Awan R, Nolan JP, Cook TM. Use of a ProSeal™ laryngeal mask airway for airway maintenance during emergency Caesarean section after failed tracheal intubation. *Br J Anaesth.* 2004; **92**: 144–6.

13 Yentis SM. The airway in obstetrics. In: Calder I, Pearce A, editors. *Core Topics in Airway Management.* Cambridge: Cambridge University Press; 2005.

14 Vadodaria BS, Gandhi SD, McIndoe AK. Comparison of four different emergency airway access equipment sets on a human patient simulator. *Anaesthesia.* 2004; **59**: 73–9.

15 Saravankumar K, Rao SG, Cooper GM. Obesity and obstetric anaesthesia. *Anaesthesia.* 2006; **61:** 36–48.

16 Department of Health and Social Security. *Report on Confidential Enquiries into Maternal Deaths in England and Wales, 1982–84. Reports on Health and Social Subjects No. 34.* London: HMSO; 1989.

17 Department of Health. *Report on Confidential Enquiries into Maternal Deaths in the United Kingdom, 1985–1987.* London: HMSO; 1991.

18 Department of Health. *Report on Confidential Enquiries into Maternal Deaths in the United Kingdom, 1988–1990.* London: HMSO; 1994.

19 Department of Health. *Report on Confidential Enquiries into Maternal Deaths in the United Kingdom, 1991–1993.* London: HMSO; 1996.

20 Department of Health. *The Confidential Enquiries into Maternal and Child Health. Why Mothers Die, 2000–2002. The Sixth Report on the Confidential Enquiries into Maternal Deaths in the United Kingdom.* London: RCOG Press; 2004.

CHAPTER 3 General anaesthesia and acid aspiration

1 Department of Health. *Reports on Confidential Enquiries into Maternal Deaths in England and Wales/United Kingdom, 1952–2002.* London: HMSO; 1957–2001 (Triennial Reports).

2 Thomas J, Paranjothy S. *National Sentinel Caesarean Section Audit Report.* London: RCOG Press; 2001.

3 Mendelson CL. Aspiration of stomach contents into lungs during obstetric anesthesia. *Am J Obstet Gynecol.* 1946; **305:** 191–206.

4 Engelhardt T, Webster NR. Pulmonary aspiration of gastric contents in anaesthesia. *Br J Anaesth.* 1999; **83:** 453–60.

5 Hawkins JL, Koonin LM, Palmer SK *et al.* Anesthesia-related deaths during obstetric delivery in the United States, 1979–1990. *Anesthesiology.* 1997; **86:** 277–84.

6 Bogod DG. The postpartum stomach – when is it safe? *Anaesthesia.* 1994; **49:** 1–2.

7 Roberts RB, Shirley MA. Reducing the risk of aspiration during caesarean section. *Anaesth Analg.* 1974; **53:** 859–68.

8 Conklin KA, Backus AM. Physiologic changes of pregnancy. In: Chestnut DH, editor. *Obstetric Anaesthesia: principles and practice.* 2nd ed. St Louis, MO: Mosby; 2004.

9 Baron TH, Ramirez B, Richter JE. Gastrointestinal motility disorders during pregnancy. *Ann Intern Med.* 1993; **118:** 366–75.

10 Sandhar BK, Elliott RH, Windram I *et al.* Peripartum changes in gastric emptying. *Anaesthesia.* 1992; **47:** 196–8.

11 Macfie AG, Magides AD, Richmond MN *et al.* Gastric emptying in pregnancy. *Br J Anaesth.* 1991; **67:** 54–7.

12 Everson GT. Gastrointestinal motility in pregnancy. *Gastroenterol Clin North Am.* 1992; **21:** 751–76.

13 Broussard CN, Richter JE. Treating gastro-oesophageal reflux disease during pregnancy and lactation. What are the safest therapy options? *Drug Safety.* 1998; **19:** 325–7.

14 Hey VM, Cowley DJ, Ganguli PC *et al.* Gastro-oesophageal reflux in late pregnancy. *Anaesthesia.* 1977; **32:** 372–7.

15 Kahrilas PJ. GERD pathogenesis, pathophysiology and clinical manifestations. *Cleve Clin J Med.* 2003: **70 (Suppl. 5):** S4–19.

16 Cotton BR, Smith G. The lower oesophageal sphincter and anaesthesia. *Br J Anaesth.* 1984; **56:** 37–46.

17 Salter RH. Lower oesophageal sphincter: therapeutic implications. *Lancet.* 1974; **7853:** 347–9.

18 Nagendran T, Nagendran S. Mechanism and treatment of nausea and vomiting. *Ala Med.* 1990; **60:** 12–16.

19 Andrews PL, Hawthorn J. The neurophysiology of vomiting. *Ballieres Clin Gastroenterol.* 1988; **2:** 141–68.

20 Naylor RJ, Inall FC. The physiology and pharmacology of postoperative nausea and vomiting. *Anaesthesia.* 1994; **49 (Suppl.):** 2–5.

21 Islam S, Jain PN. Post-operative nausea and vomiting (PONV): a review article. *Indian J Anaesth.* 2004; **48:** 253–8.

22 Hey VM, Ostick DG. Metoclopramide and the gastro-oesophageal sphincter. A study in pregnant women with heartburn. *Anaesthesia.* 1978; **33:** 462–5.

23 Brock-Utne JG. Metoclopramide and the gastro-oesophageal sphincter. *Anaesthesia.* 1979; **34:** 81–3.

24 Lopez-Olaondo L, Carrascosa F, Puevo FJ *et al.* Combination of ondansetron and dexamethasone in the prophylaxis of postoperative nausea and vomiting. *Br J Anaesth.* 1996; **76:** 835–40.

25 Moore J, Flynn RJ, Sampaio M *et al.* Effect of single-dose omeprazole on intragastric acidity and volume during obstetric anaesthesia. *Anaesthesia.* 1989; **44:** 559–62.

26 Hirota K, Kushikata T. Pre-anaesthetic H_2 antagonists for acid aspiration pneumonia prophylaxis. Is there evidence of tolerance? *Br J Anaesth.* 2003; **90:** 576–9.

27 Calthorpe N, Lewis M. Acid aspiration prophylaxis in labour: a survey of UK obstetric units. *Int J Obstet Anesth.* 2005; **14:** 300–4.

28 Grieff JMC, Tordoff SG, Griffiths R *et al.* Acid aspiration prophylaxis in 202 obstetric anaesthetic units in the UK. *Int J Obstet Anesth.* 1994; **3:** 137–42.

29 Ginosar Y, Russell IF, Halpern SH. Is regional anaesthesia safer than general anaesthesia for caesarean section? In: Halpern SH, Douglas MJ, editors. *Evidence-Based Obstetric Anaesthesia.* Oxford: Blackwell Publishing; 2005.

30 O'Sullivan GO, Hart D, Shennan A. A rational approach to aspiration prophylaxis. In: Halpern SH, Douglas MJ, editors. *Evidence-Based Obstetric Anaesthesia.* Oxford: Blackwell Publishing; 2005.

CHAPTER 4 Regional anaesthesia

1 Collier CB. Total spinal or massive subdural block? *Anaesth Intensive Care.* 1982; **10:** 92–3.

2 Collier CB. Accidental subdural injection during attempted lumbar epidural block may present as a failed or inadequate block: radiographic evidence. *Reg Anesth Pain Med.* 2004; **29:** 45–51.

3 Albright GA. Cardiac arrest following regional anesthesia with etidocaine or bupivacaine. *Anesthesiology.* 1979; **51:** 285–6.

4 Hawkins JL, Koonin LM, Palmer SK *et al.* Anesthesia-related deaths during obstetric delivery in the United States, 1979–1990. *Anesthesiology.* 1997; **86:** 277–84.

5 Department of Health and Social Security. *Report on Confidential Enquiries into Maternal Deaths in England and Wales, 1982–84. Reports on Health and Social Subjects No. 34.* London: HMSO; 1989.

6 Department of Health. *Report on Confidential Enquiries into Maternal Deaths in the United Kingdom, 1985–1987.* London: HMSO; 1991.

7 Milligan KR, Carp H. Continuous spinal anesthesia for caesarean section in the morbidly obese. *Int J Obstet Anesth.* 1992; **1**: 111–13.

8 Gardner IC, Kinsella SM. Obstetric epidural test doses: a survey of UK practice. *Int J Obstet Anesth.* 2005; **14**: 96–103.

9 Department of Health. *Report on Confidential Enquiries into Maternal Deaths in the United Kingdom, 1988–1990.* London: HMSO; 1994.

10 Department of Health. *Why Mothers Die, 1997–1999. The Fifth Report on the Confidential Enquiries into Maternal Deaths in the United Kingdom.* London: RCOG Press; 2001.

11 Department of Health. *Why Mothers Die, 2000–2002. The Sixth Report on the Confidential Enquiries into Maternal Deaths in the United Kingdom.* London: RCOG Press; 2004; www.cemach.org.uk

12 Wahl A, Eberli FR, Thomson DA *et al.* Coronary artery spasm and non-Q-wave myocardial infarction following intravenous ephedrine in two healthy women under spinal anaesthesia. *Br J Anaesth.* 2002; **89**: 519–23.

13 Riley ET. Spinal anaesthesia for Caesarean delivery: keep the pressure up and don't spare the vasoconstrictors. *Br J Anaesth.* 2004; **92**: 459–61.

14 MacLennan FM. Maternal mortality from Mendelson's syndrome: an explanation? *Lancet.* 1986; **1**: 587–9.

15 Department of Health. *Report on Confidential Enquiries into Maternal Deaths in the United Kingdom, 1991–1993.* London: HMSO; 1996.

16 Department of Health. *Why Mothers Die. Report on the Confidential Enquiries into Maternal Deaths in the United Kingdom, 1994–96.* London: The Stationery Office; 1998.

17 Mardirosoff C, Dumont L, Lemedioni P *et al.* Sensory block extension during combined spinal and epidural. *Reg Anesth Pain Med.* 1998; **23**: 92–5.

18 Reynolds F. Damage to the conus medullaris following spinal anaesthesia. *Anaesthesia.* 2001; **56**: 238–47.

19 Myint Y, Bailey PW, Milne BR. Cardiorespiratory arrest following combined spinal epidural anaesthesia for Caesarean section. *Anaesthesia.* 1993; **48**: 684–6.

20 Kinsella SM, Tuckey JP. Perioperative bradycardia and asystole: relationship to vasovagal syncope and the Bezold–Jarisch reflex. *Br J Anaesth.* 2001; **86**: 859–68.

21 Rosenberg JM, Wahr JA, Sung CH *et al.* Coronary perfusion pressure during cardiopulmonary resuscitation after spinal anesthesia in dogs. *Anesth Analg.* 1996; **82**: 84–7.

22 Department of Health. *Why Mothers Die, 1997–1999. The Fifth Report on the Confidential Enquiries into Maternal Deaths in the United Kingdom.* London: RCOG Press; 2001.

23 Laishley R. In the event of accidental dural puncture by an epidural needle in labour, the catheter should be passed into the subarachnoid space (opposer). *Int J Obstet Anesth.* 2002; **11**: 26–7.

24 McBrien ME, Bali IM. Untoward incident reporting in obstetric anaesthesia: a 6-month prospective study in Northern Ireland. *Int J Obstet Anesth.* 1996; **5**: 225–8.

25 Shibli KU, Russell IF. A survey of anaesthetic techniques used for caesarean section in the UK in 1997. *Int J Obstet Anesth.* 2000; **9**: 160–7.

26 Paech MJ, Godkin R, Webster S. Complications of obstetric epidural analgesia and anaesthesia: a prospective analysis of 10,995 cases. *Int J Obstet Anesth.* 1998; **7**: 5–11.

27 Kar GS, Jenkins JG. High spinal anaesthesia: two cases encountered in a survey of 81,322 obstetric epidurals. *Int J Obstet Anesth.* 2001; **10**: 189–91.

28 Crawford JS. Some maternal complications of epidural analgesia in labour. *Anaesthesia.* 1985; **40**: 1219–52.

29 Van Zundert A, Wolfe AM, Vaes L *et al.* High-volume spinal anesthesia with bupivacaine 0.125% for Cesarean section. *Anesthesiology.* 1988; **69**: 998–1003.

30 Kinsella SM. Lateral tilt for pregnant women: why 15 degrees? *Anaesthesia.* 2003; **58**: 835–7.

31 Russell R, Popat M, Richards E *et al.* Combined spinal epidural anaesthesia for caesarean section: a randomised comparison of Oxford, lateral and sitting positions. *Int J Obstet Anesth.* 2002; **11**: 190–5.

32 Vucevic M, Russell IF. Spinal anaesthesia for caesarean section: 0.125% plain bupivacaine 12 ml compared with 0.5% plain bupivacaine 3 ml. *Br J Anaesth.* 1992; **68**: 590–5.

33 Russell IF. Total spinal or massive subdural? *Anaesth Intensive Care.* 1983; **11**: 386–7.

34 Bonica JJ, Berges PU, Morikawa K. Circulatory effects of peridural block. I. Effects of level of analgesia and dose of lidocaine. *Anesthesiology.* 1970; **33**: 619–26.

35 Bonica JJ, Kennedy WF, Akamatsu TJ *et al.* Circulatory effects of peridural block. III. Effects of acute blood loss. *Anesthesiology.* 1972; **36**: 219–27.

36 Kopp SL, Horlocker TT, Warner ME *et al.* Cardiac arrest during neuraxial anesthesia: frequency and predisposing factors associated with survival. *Anesth Analg.* 2005; **100**: 855–65.

37 Caplan RA, Ward RJ, Posner K *et al.* Unexpected cardiac arrest during spinal anesthesia: a closed claims analysis of predisposing factors. *Anesthesiology.* 1988; **68**: 5–11.

38 Rees GAD, Willis BA. Resuscitation in late pregnancy. *Anaesthesia.* 1988; **43**: 347–9.

39 www.erc.edu/index.php/guidelines

40 Emmett RS, Cyna AM, Andrew M *et al.* Techniques for preventing hypotension during spinal anaesthesia for caesarean section. *The Cochrane Database of Systematic Reviews. Issue 3.* Oxford: Update Software; 2002.

41 Rout CC, Akoojee SS, Rocke DA *et al.* Rapid administration of crystalloid preload does not decrease the incidence of hypotension after spinal anaesthesia for elective Caesarean section. *Br J Anaesth.* 1992; **68**: 394–7.

42 Dyer RA, Farina Z, Joubert IA *et al.* Crystalloid prehydration versus rapid crystalloid administration after induction of spinal ananesthesia (coload) for elective caesarean section. *Anaesth Intensive Care.* 2004; **2**: 351–7.

43 Ngan Kee WD, Khaw KS, Ng FF. Prevention of hypotension during spinal anesthesia for caesarean delivery. An effective technique using combination phenylephrine infusion and crystalloid cohydration. *Anesthesiology.* 2005; **103**: 744–50.

44 Burns SM, Cowan CM, Wilkes RG. Prevention and management of hypotension during spinal anaesthesia for elective Caesarean section: a survey of practice. *Anaesthesia.* 2001; **56**: 794–8.

45 Shnider SM, De Lormier AA, Holl JW *et al.* Vasopressors in obstetrics: correction of fetal acidosis with ephedrine during spinal hypotension. *Am J Obstet Gynecol.* 1968; **102**: 911–19.

46 Lee A, Ngan Kee WD, Gin T. A quantitative, systematic review of randomized controlled trials of ephedrine versus phenylephrine for the management of hypotension during spinal anesthesia for cesarean delivery. *Anesth Analg.* 2002; **94**: 920–6.

47 Lee A, Ngan Kee WD, Gin T. A dose–response meta-analysis of prophylactic intravenous ephedrine for the prevention of hypotension during spinal anesthesia for elective cesarean delivery. *Anesth Analg.* 2004; **98**: 483–90.

48 Ngan Kee WD, Khaw KS, Ng FF. Comparison of phenylephrine infusion regimens for maintaining maternal blood pressure during spinal anaesthesia for Caesarean section. *Br J Anaesth.* 2004; **92**: 469–74.

49 Yentis SM, Dob DP. High regional block – the failed intubation of the new millennium? *Int J Obstet Anesth.* 2001; **10:** 159–61.

CHAPTER 5 Haemorrhage

1 Drife J. Management of primary postpartum haemorrhage. *Br J Obstet Gynaecol.* 1997; **104:** 275–7.

2 Chang AB. Physiological changes of pregnancy. In: Chestnut DH, editor. *Obstetric Anaesthesia: principles and practice.* 3rd ed. Philadelphia, PA: Elsevier Mosby; 2004. pp. 15–36.

3 Seeley H. Massive blood loss in obstetrics. In: Chamberlain G, editor. *Turnbull's Obstetrics.* 2nd ed. Edinburgh: Churchill Livingstone; 1995. pp. 735–45.

4 Mayer DC, Spielman FJ, Bell EA. Antepartum and postpartum haemorrhage. In: Chestnut DH, editor. *Obstetric Anaesthesia: principles and practice.* 3rd ed. Philadelphia, PA: Elsevier Mosby; 2004. pp. 662–82.

5 Holdcroft A, Thomas TA. *Principles and Practice of Obstetric Anaesthesia and Analgesia.* Oxford: Blackwell Science; 2000.

6 Department of Health. Antepartum and postpartum haemorrhage. In: *Why Mothers Die. Report on the Confidential Enquiries into Maternal Deaths in the United Kingdom, 1994–96.* London: The Stationery Office; 1998. pp. 47–56.

7 Department of Health. Anaesthesia. In: *Why Mothers Die, 1997–1999. The Fifth Report on the Confidential Enquiries into Maternal Deaths in the United Kingdom.* London: RCOG Press; 2001. pp. 134–49.

8 Tulandi T, Al-Jaroudi D. Interstitial pregnancy: results generated from the Society of Reproductive Surgeons registry. *Obstet Gynecol.* 2004; **103:** 47–50.

9 Department of Health. Haemorrhage. In: *Why Mothers Die, 1997–1999. The Fifth Report on the Confidential Enquiries into Maternal Deaths in the United Kingdom.* London: RCOG Press; 2001. pp. 94–103.

10 Kuczkowski KM. Cocaine abuse in pregnancy – anesthetic implications. *Int J Obstet Anesth.* 2002; **11:** 204–10.

11 Department of Health. Genital tract trauma. In: *Report on Confidential Enquiries into Maternal Deaths in the United Kingdom, 1991–1993.* London: HMSO; 1996. pp. 84–6.

12 Kamani AA, McMorland GH, Wadsworth LD. Utilisation of red blood cell transfusion in an obstetric setting. *Am J Obstet Gynecol.* 1988; **159:** 1177–81.

13 B-Lynch C, Coker A, Lawal AH *et al.* The B-Lynch surgical technique for the control of massive postpartum haemorrhage: an alternative to hysterectomy? Five cases reported. *Br J Obstet Gynaecol.* 1997; **104:** 372–5.

14 Department of Health. Antepartum and postpartum haemorrhage. In: *Report on Confidential Enquiries into Maternal Deaths in the United Kingdom, 1991–1993.* London: HMSO; 1996. pp. 32–43.

15 Department of Health. Guidelines for the management and treatment of obstetric haemorrhage in women who decline blood transfusion. In: *Why Mothers Die, 2000–2002. The Sixth Report on the Confidential Enquiries into Maternal Deaths in the United Kingdom.* London: RCOG Press; 2004. pp. 94–5.

16 Norman KE. Alternative treatments for disseminated intravascular coagulation. *Drug News Perspect.* 2004; **17:** 243–50.

17 Sharma SK, Lechner RB. Hematologic and coagulation disorders. In: Chestnut DH, editor. *Obstetric Anaesthesia: principles and practice.* 3rd ed. Philadelphia, PA: Elsevier Mosby; 2004. pp. 764–79.

18 Levi M. Disseminated intravascular coagulation: what's new? *Crit Care Clin.* 2005; **21**: 449–67.

19 Department of Health. Genital tract trauma and other direct deaths. In: *Why Mothers Die, 1997–1999. The Fifth Report of the Confidential Enquiries into Maternal Deaths in the United Kingdom.* London: RCOG Press; 2001. pp. 130–3.

20 Department of Health. Haemorrhage. In: *The Confidential Enquiries into Maternal and Child Health. Why Mothers Die, 2000–2002. The Sixth Report on the Confidential Enquiries into Maternal Deaths in the United Kingdom.* London: RCOG Press; 2004. pp. 86–93.

21 Shevell T, Malone FD. Management of obstetric haemorrhage. *Semin Perinatol.* 2003; **27**: 86–104.

22 Banks A, Norris A. Massive haemorrhage in pregnancy. *Cont Educ Anaesth Crit Care Pain.* 2005; **5**: 195–8.

23 McClelland DBL. *Handbook of Transfusion Medicine.* 3rd ed. London: The Stationery Office; 2001.

24 Department of Health. Revised guidelines for the management of massive obstetric haemorrhage. In: *Report on the Confidential Enquiries into Maternal Deaths in the United Kingdom, 1988–1990.* London: HMSO; 1994. pp. 43–4.

25 Spahn DR, Rossaint R. Coagulopathy and blood component transfusion in trauma. *Br J Anaesth.* 2005; **95**: 130–9.

26 Ahonen J, Jokela R. Recombinant factor VIIa for life-threatening post-partum haemorrhage. *Br J Anaesth.* 2005; **94**: 592–5.

27 National Institute for Clinical Excellence. *Guidance on the Use of Ultrasound Devices for Placing Central Venous Catheters.* London: National Institute for Clinical Excellence; 2002.

28 Department of Health. Deaths associated with anaesthesia. In: *Report on Confidential Enquiries into Maternal Deaths in the United Kingdom, 1991–1993.* London: HMSO; 1996. pp. 87–102.

29 National Institute for Clinical Excellence. *Intraoperative Blood Cell Salvage in Obstetrics.* London: National Institute for Clinical Excellence; 2005.

30 As AK, Hagen P, Webb JB. Tranexamic acid in the management of postpartum haemorrhage. *Br J Obstet Gynaecol.* 1996; **103**: 1250–1.

31 Svanberg L, Astedt B, Nilsson IM. Abruptio placentae – treatment with fibrinolytic inhibitor tranexamic acid. *Acta Obstet Gynecol Scand.* 1980; **59**: 127–30.

32 Valentine S, Williamson P, Sutton D. Reduction of acute haemorrhage with aprotinin. *Anaesthesia.* 1993; **48**: 405–6.

33 Sher G. Trasylol in the management of abruptio placentae with consumption coagulopathy and uterine inertia. *J Reprod Med.* 1980; **25**: 113–18.

CHAPTER 6 Hypertension

1 Fox H. Pathology of the placenta. *Clin Obstet Gynaecol.* 1986; **13**: 501–19.

2 Spaanderman M, Ekhart T, van Eyck J *et al.* Pre-eclampsia and maladaptation to pregnancy: a role for atrial natriuretic peptide? *Kidney Int.* 2001; **60**: 1397–406.

3 Roberts JM. Pre-eclampsia: what we know and what we do not know. *Semin Perinatol.* 2000; **24**: 24–8.

4 Department of Health. *Why Mothers Die, 2000–2002. The Sixth Report on the Confidential Enquiries into Maternal Deaths in the United Kingdom.* London: RCOG Press; 2004.

5 Department of Health. *Why Mothers Die, 1997–99. The Fifth Report on the Confidential Enquiries into Maternal Deaths in the United Kingdom.* London: RCOG Press; 2001.

6 Natarajan P, Shennan AH, Penny J *et al.* Comparison of auscultatory and oscillometric automated blood pressure monitors in the setting of pre-eclampsia. *Am J Obstet Gynecol.* 1999; **181:** 1203–10.

7 Golara M, Benedict A, Jones C *et al.* Inflationary oscillometry provides accurate measurement of blood pressure in pre-eclampsia. *Br J Obstet Gynaecol.* 2002; **109:** 1143–7.

8 Department of Health. *Report on Confidential Enquiries into Maternal Deaths in the United Kingdom, 1988–1990.* London: HMSO; 1994.

9 Magee LA, Cham C, Waterman EJ *et al.* Hydralazine for treatment of severe hypertension in pregnancy: meta-analysis. *BMJ.* 2003; **327:** 955–60.

10 Shnider SM, Abboud TK, Artal R *et al.* Maternal catecholamines decrease during labor after lumbar epidural anesthesia. *Am J Obstet Gynecol.* 1983; **147:** 13–15.

11 The Eclampsia Trial Collaborative Group. Which anticonvulsant for women with eclampsia? Evidence from the Collaborative Eclampsia Trial. *Lancet.* 1995; **345:** 1455–63.

12 Wee L, Sinha P, Lewis M. The management of eclampsia by obstetric anaesthetists in UK: a postal survey. *Int J Obstet Anesth.* 2001; **10:** 108–12.

13 Royal College of Obstetricians and Gynaecologists. *Management of Eclampsia. Guideline No. 10(A).* London: Royal College of Obstetricians and Gynaecologists; 2006.

14 Holdcroft A, Oatridge A, Fusi L *et al.* Magnetic resonance imaging in preeclampsia and eclampsia complicated by visual disturbance and other neurological abnormalities. *Int J Obstet Anesth.* 2002; **11:** 255–9.

15 The Magpie Trial Collaborative Group. Do women with pre-eclampsia, and their babies, benefit from magnesium sulphate? The Magpie trial: a randomised placebo-controlled trial. *Lancet.* 2002; **359:** 1877–90.

16 Department of Health. *Report on Confidential Enquiries into Maternal Deaths in the United Kingdom, 1985–1987.* London: HMSO; 1991.

17 Department of Health. *Why Mothers Die. Report on the Confidential Enquiries into Maternal Deaths in the United Kingdom, 1994–96.* London: The Stationery Office; 1998.

18 Barry C, Fox R, Stirrat G. Upper abdominal pain in pregnancy may indicate pre-eclampsia. *BMJ.* 1994; **308:** 1562–3.

19 Gonik B, Cotton D, Spillman T *et al.* Peripartum colloid osmotic pressure changes: effects of controlled fluid management. *Am J Obstet Gynecol.* 1985; **151:** 812–15.

20 Engelhardt T, MacLennan FM. Fluid management in pre-eclampsia. *Int J Obstet Anesth.* 1999; **8:** 253–9.

21 Park GE, Hauch MA, Curlin F *et al.* The effects of varying volumes of crystalloid administration before cesarean delivery on maternal hemodynamics and colloid osmotic pressure. *Anesth Analg.* 1996; **83:** 299–303.

22 Benedetti TJ, Kates R, Williams V. Hemodynamic observations in severe pre-eclampsia complicated by pulmonary edema. *Am J Obstet Gynecol.* 1985; **152:** 330–4.

23 Shoemaker WC, Appel PL, Kram HB *et al.* Prospective trial of supranormal values of survivors as therapeutic goals in high-risk surgical patients. *Chest.* 1988; **94:** 1176–86.

24 Kramer RL, Van Someren JK, Qualls CR *et al.* Postoperative management of cesarean patients: the effect of immediate feeding on the incidence of ileus. *Obstet Gynecol.* 1996; **88:** 29–32.

25 Department of Health. *Report on Confidential Enquiries into Maternal Deaths in the United Kingdom, 1991–1993.* London: HMSO; 1996.

26 National Institute for Clinical Excellence. *Full Guidance on the Use of Ultrasound Locating Devices for Placing Central Venous Catheters.* Technology Appraisal Guidance No. 49. London: National Institute for Clinical Excellence; 2002.

27 Harvey S, Harrison DA, Singer M *et al.* Assessment of the clinical effectiveness of pulmonary artery catheters in the management of critically ill patients in intensive care (PAC-Man): a randomised controlled trial. *Lancet.* 2005; **366**: 472–7.

28 Chittock DR, Dhingra VK, Ronco JJ *et al.* Severity of illness and risk of death associated with pulmonary artery catheter use. *Crit Care Med.* 2004; **32**: 911–15.

29 Cotton DB, Gonik B, Dorman K *et al.* Cardiovascular alterations in severe pregnancy-induced hypertension: relationship of central venous pressure to pulmonary capillary wedge pressure. *Am J Obstet Gynecol.* 1985; **151**: 762–4.

30 Cotton DB, Lee W, Huhta JC *et al.* Hemodynamic profile of severe pregnancy-induced hypertension. *Am J Obstet Gynecol.* 1988; **158**: 523–9.

31 National Collaborating Centre for Women's and Children's Health, commissioned by National Institute for Clinical Excellence. *Caesarean Section: clinical guideline.* London: RCOG Press; 2004.

32 Prys-Roberts C. Phaeochromocytoma – recent advances in its management. *Br J Anaesth.* 2000; **85**: 44–57.

CHAPTER 7 Cardiac disease

1 Department of Health. *Why Mothers Die, 2000–2002. The Sixth Report on the Confidential Enquiries into Maternal Deaths in the United Kingdom.* London: RCOG Press; 2004.

2 Uebing A, Steer PJ, Yentis SM *et al.* Pregnancy and congenital heart disease. *BMJ.* 2006; **332**: 401–6.

3 Department of Health. *Why Mothers Die, 1997–1999. The Fifth Report on the Confidential Enquiries into Maternal Deaths in the United Kingdom.* London: RCOG Press; 2001.

4 Warnes CA. Pregnancy and pulmonary hypertension. *Int J Cardiol.* 2004; **97**: 11–13.

5 Mangano DT. Anesthesia for the pregnant cardiac patient. In: Hughes S, Levinson G, Rosen M, editors. *Anesthesia for Obstetrics.* 4th ed. Philadelphia, PA: Lippincott Williams & Wilkins; 2002. pp. 455–95.

6 Weiss BM, Zemp L, Seifert B *et al.* Outcome of pulmonary vascular disease in pregnancy: a systematic overview from 1978–1996. *J Am Coll Cardiol.* 1998; **31**: 1650–7.

7 Dob DP, Yentis SM. Practical management of the parturient with congenital heart disease. *Int J Obstet Anesth.* 2006; **15**: 137–44.

8 Bonnin M, Mercier FJ, Sitbon O *et al.* Severe pulmonary hypertension during pregnancy. *Anesthesiology.* 2005; **102**: 1133–7.

9 Khan MJ, Bhatt SB, Krye JJ. Anesthetic consideration for parturients with primary pulmonary hypertension: review of the literature and clinical presentation. *Int J Obstet Anesth.* 1996; **5**: 36–42.

10 Khan IA, Nair CK. Clinical, diagnostic and management perspectives of aortic dissection. *Chest.* 2002; **122**: 311–28.

11 Lewis S, Ryder I, Lovell AT. Peripartum presentation of an acute aortic dissection. *Br J Anaesth.* 2005; **94**: 496–9.

12 Ray P, Murphy GJ, Shutt LE. Recognition and management of maternal cardiac disease in pregnancy. *Br J Anaesth.* 2004; **93**: 428–39.

13 Weissmann-Brenner A, Schoen R, Divon MY. Aortic dissection in pregnancy. *Obstet Gynecol.* 2004; **103**: 1110–13.

14 Zeebregts CJ, Schepens MA, Hameeteman TM *et al.* Acute aortic dissection complicating pregnancy. *Ann Thorac Surg.* 1997; **64**: 1345–8.

15 de Swiet M. Cardiac deaths. In: MacLean AB, Neilson JP, editors. *Maternal Morbidity and Mortality*. London: RCOG Press; 2002. pp. 259–70.

16 Badhi E, Enciso R. Acute myocardial infarction during pregnancy and puerperium: a review. *Angiology*. 1996; **47**: 739–56.

17 Siu SC, Sermer M, Coleman JM *et al*. Prospective multicenter study of pregnancy outcomes in women with heart disease. *Circulation*. 2001; **104**: 515–21.

18 Head CEG, Thorne SA. Congenital heart disease in pregnancy. *Postgrad Med J*. 2005; **81**: 292–8.

19 Thorne SA. Pregnancy in heart disease. *Heart*. 2004; **90**: 450–6.

20 Horlocker TT, Wedel DJ, Benzon H *et al*. Regional anesthesia in the anticoagulated patient: defining the risks. *Reg Anesth Pain Med*. 2003; **28**: 172–97.

21 Pinder AJ, Dresner M, Calow C *et al*. Haemodynamic changes caused by oxytocin during caesarean section under spinal anaesthesia. *Int J Obstet Anesth*. 2002; **11**: 156–9.

22 Royal College of Obstetricians and Gynaecologists. *Thromboprophylaxis During Pregnancy, Labour and After Vaginal Delivery*. RCOG Guideline No. 37. London: Royal College of Obstetricians and Gynaecologists; www.rcog.org.uk/resources/Public/pdf/Thromboprophylaxis_no037.pdf

23 Orme RMLE, Grange CS, Ainsworth QP *et al*. General anaesthesia using remifentanil for caesarean section in parturients with critical aortic stenosis. *Int J Obstet Anesth*. 2004; **13**: 183–7.

24 Dob DP, Yentis SM. UK registry of high-risk obstetric anaesthesia: report on cardiorespiratory disease. *Int J Obstet Anesth*. 2001; **10**: 267–72.

25 Johanson R, Cox C, Grady K and Howell C, editors. *Managing Obstetric Emergencies and Trauma*. London: RCOG Press; 2003.

26 www.also.org.uk/courses.asp (accessed 10 January 2007).

CHAPTER 8A Thromboembolism

1 Department of Health. *Why Mothers Die, 2000–2002. The Sixth Report on the Confidential Enquiries into Maternal Deaths in the United Kingdom*. London: RCOG Press; 2004.

2 Eldor A. Thrombophilia, thrombosis and pregnancy. *Thromb Haemost*. 2001; **86**: 104–11.

3 Grendys EC Jr, Fiorica JV. Advances in the prevention and treatment of deep vein thrombosis and pulmonary embolism. *Curr Opin Obstet Gynecol*. 1999; **11**: 71–9.

4 Macklon NS, Greer IA. Venous thromboembolic disease in obstetrics and gynaecology: the Scottish experience. *Scott Med J*. 1996; **41**: 83–6.

5 Greer IA. Thrombosis in pregnancy: maternal and fetal issues. *Lancet*. 1999; **353**: 1258–65.

6 McColl MD, Ramsay JE, Tait RC *et al*. Risk factors for pregnancy-associated venous thromboembolism. *Thromb Haemost*. 1997; **78**: 1183–8.

7 Ray JG, Chan WS. Deep vein thrombosis during pregnancy and the puerperium: a meta-analysis of the period of risk and the leg of presentation. *Obstet Gynecol Surv*. 1999; **54**: 265–71.

8 Gherman RB, Goodwin TM, Leung B *et al*. Incidence, clinical characteristics, and timing of objectively diagnosed venous thromboembolism during pregnancy. *Obstet Gynecol*. 1999; **94**: 730–4.

9 Greer IA. The acute management of venous thromboembolism in pregnancy. *Curr Opin Obstet Gynecol*. 2001; **13**: 569–75.

10 Department of Health. *Why Mothers Die, 1997–1999. The Fifth Report on the Confidential Enquiries into Maternal Deaths in the United Kingdom*. London: RCOG Press; 2001.

11 Macklon NS, Greer IA, Bowman AW. An ultrasound study of gestational and postural changes in the deep venous system of the leg in pregnancy. *Br J Obstet Gynaecol.* 1997; **104**: 191–7.

12 Lockwood CJ. Inherited thrombophilias in pregnant patients: detection and treatment paradigm. *Obstet Gynecol.* 2002; **99**: 333–41.

13 Kupferminc MJ. Thrombophilia and pregnancy. *Reprod Biol Endocrinol.* 2003; **1**: 111.

14 Greer IA. Inherited thrombophilia and venous thromboembolism. *Best Pract Res Clin Obstet Gynaecol.* 2003; **17**: 413–25.

15 McLintock C, North RA, Dekker G. Inherited thrombophilias: associated venous thromboembolism and obstetric complications. *Curr Probl Obstet Gynecol Fertil.* 2001; **24**: 109–52.

16 Friederich PW, Sanson BJ, Simioni P *et al.* Frequency of pregnancy-related venous thromboembolism in anticoagulant factor-deficient women: implications for prophylaxis. *Ann Intern Med.* 1996; **125**: 955–60.

17 Eichinger S, Stumpflen A, Hirschl M *et al.* Hyperhomocysteinemia is a risk factor of recurrent venous thromboembolism. *Thromb Haemost.* 1998; **80**: 566–9.

18 Robertson L, Wu O, Langhorne P *et al.* The Thrombosis Risk and Economic Assessment of Thrombophilia Screening (TREATS) Study. Thrombophilia in pregnancy: a systematic review. *Br J Haematol.* 2006; **132**: 171–96.

19 Robertson L, Greer I. Thromboembolism in pregnancy. *Curr Opin Obstet Gynecol.* 2005; **17**: 113–16.

20 Hague WM, Dekker GA. Risk factors for thrombosis in pregnancy. *Best Pract Res Clin Haematol.* 2003; **16**: 197–210.

21 Khamashta MA, Cuadrado MJ, Mujic F *et al.* The management of thrombosis in the antiphospholipid-antibody syndrome. *NEJM.* 1995; **332**: 993–7.

22 Gherman RB, Goodwin TM, Leung B *et al.* Incidence, clinical characteristics, and timing of objectively diagnosed venous thromboembolism during pregnancy. *Obstet Gynecol.* 1999; **94**: 730–4.

23 Brill-Edwards P, Ginsberg JS, Gent M *et al.* Safety of withholding heparin in pregnant women with a history of venous thromboembolism. Recurrence of clot in this pregnancy study group. *NEJM.* 2000; **343**: 1439–44.

24 Lensing AW, Prandoni P, Brandjes D *et al.* Detection of deep-vein thrombosis by real-time B-mode ultrasonography. *NEJM.* 1989; **320**: 342–5.

25 Tapson VF, Carroll BA, Davidson BL *et al.* The diagnostic approach to acute venous thromboembolism. American Thoracic Society clinical practice guidelines. *Am J Respir Crit Care Med.* 1999; **160**: 1043–66.

26 Fraser DG, Moody AR, Morgan PS *et al.* Diagnosis of lower-limb deep venous thrombosis: a prospective blinded study of magnetic resonance direct thrombus imaging. *Ann Intern Med.* 2002; **136**: 89–98.

27 Nijkeuter M, Ginsberg JS, Huisman MV. Diagnosis of deep vein thrombosis and pulmonary embolism in pregnancy: a systematic review. *J Thromb Haemost.* 2006; **4**: 496–500.

28 Lumb A. *Nunn's Applied Respiratory Physiology.* 6th ed. Oxford: Elsevier Butterworth-Heinemann; 2005. pp. 393–5.

29 Malinow A. Embolic disorders. In: Chestnut D, editor. *Obstetric Anesthesia: principles and practice.* 3rd ed. Philadelphia, PA: Elsevier Mosby; 2004. pp. 683–8.

30 Spence TH. Pulmonary embolization syndrome. In: Civetta JM, Taylor RM, Kirby RR, editors. *Critical Care.* Philadelphia, PA: JB Lippincott; 1988. pp. 1091–102.

31 Ginsberg JS, Hirsh J, Rainbow AJ *et al*. Risks to the fetus of radiologic procedures used in the diagnosis of maternal venous thromboembolic disease. *Thromb Haemost*. 1989; **61**: 189–96.

32 Wheeler HB, Hirsh J, Wells P *et al*. Diagnostic tests for deep vein thrombosis. Clinical usefulness depends on probability of disease. *Arch Intern Med*. 1994; **154**: 1921–8.

33 Chan WS, Ginsberg JS. Diagnosis of deep vein thrombosis and pulmonary embolism in pregnancy. *Thromb Res*. 2002; **107**: 85–91.

34 Chan WS, Chunilal SD, Lee AY *et al*. Diagnosis of deep vein thrombosis during pregnancy: a pilot study evaluating the role of d-dimer and compression leg ultrasound during pregnancy. *Blood*. 2002; **100**: 275a.

35 Donaldson J. Neurological disorders. In: de Swiet M, editor. *Medical Disorders in Obstetric Practice*. 4th ed. Oxford: Blackwell Science; 2002. pp. 490–91.

36 Chan WS, Anand S, Ginsberg JS. Anticoagulation of pregnant women with mechanical heart valves: a systematic review of the literature. *Arch Intern Med*. 2000; **160**: 191–6.

37 Sanson BJ, Lensing AW, Prins MH *et al*. Safety of low-molecular-weight heparin in pregnancy: a systematic review. *Thromb Haemost*. 1999; **81**: 668–72.

38 Chunilal SD, Young E, Johnston MA *et al*. The APTT response of pregnant plasma to unfractionated heparin. *Thromb Haemost*. 2002; **87**: 92–7.

39 Hommes DW, Bura A, Mazzolai L *et al*. Subcutaneous heparin compared with continuous intravenous heparin administration in the initial treatment of deep vein thrombosis. A meta-analysis. *Ann Intern Med*. 1992; **116**: 279–84.

40 Dolovich LR, Ginsberg JS, Douketis JD *et al*. A meta-analysis comparing low-molecular-weight heparins with unfractionated heparin in the treatment of venous thromboembolism: examining some unanswered questions regarding location of treatment, product type, and dosing frequency. *Arch Intern Med*. 2000; **160**: 181–8.

41 de Valk HW, Banga JD, Wester JW *et al*. Comparing subcutaneous danaparoid with intravenous unfractionated heparin for the treatment of venous thromboembolism. A randomized controlled trial. *Ann Intern Med*. 1995; **123**: 1–9.

42 Ginsberg JS, Bates SM. Management of venous thromboembolism during pregnancy. *J Thromb Haemost*. 2003; **1**: 1435–42.

43 Holst J, Lindblad B, Bergqvist D *et al*. Protamine neutralization of intravenous and subcutaneous low-molecular-weight heparin (tinzaparin, Logiparin). An experimental investigation in healthy volunteers. *Blood Coagul Fibrinolysis*. 1994; **5**: 795–803.

44 Tapson VF, Witty LA. Massive pulmonary embolism. Diagnostic and therapeutic strategies. *Clin Chest Med*. 1995; **16**: 329–40.

45 Douketis JD, Ginsberg JS, Burrows RF *et al*. The effects of long-term heparin therapy during pregnancy on bone density. A prospective matched cohort study. *Thromb Haemost*. 1996; **75**: 254–7.

46 Warkentin TE, Levine MN, Hirsh J *et al*. Heparin-induced thrombocytopenia in patients treated with low-molecular-weight heparin or unfractionated heparin. *NEJM*. 1995; **32**: 1330–5.

47 Royal College of Obstetricians and Gynaecologists. *Thromboprophylaxis During Pregnancy, Labour and After Vaginal Delivery. Guideline No. 37*. London: RCOG Press; 2004.

CHAPTER 8B Amniotic fluid embolism

1 Meyer JR. Embolia pulmonar amnio-caseosa. *Brasil Med*. 1926; **2**: 301–3.

2 Steiner PE, Lushbaugh CC. Maternal pulmonary embolism by amniotic fluid as a cause of obstetric shock and unexpected deaths in obstetrics. *JAMA*. 1986; **255**: 2187–203.

3 Martin RW. Amniotic fluid embolism. *Clin Obstet Gynecol*. 1996; **39**: 101–6.

4 Kelly MC, Bailie K, McCourt KC. A case of amniotic fluid embolism in a twin pregnancy in the second trimester. *Int J Obstet Anesth*. 1995; **4**: 175–7.

5 Olcott C 4th, Robinson AJ, Maxwell TM *et al*. Amniotic fluid embolism and disseminated intravascular coagulation after blunt abdominal trauma. *J Trauma*. 1973; **13**: 737–40.

6 Tramoni G, Valentin S, Robert MO *et al*. Amniotic fluid embolism during caesarean section. *Int J Obstet Anesth*. 2005; **13**: 271–4.

7 Gilbert WM, Danielsen B. Amniotic fluid embolism: decreased mortality in a population-based study. *Obstet Gynecol*. 1999; **93**: 973–7.

8 Clark SL, Hankins GD, Dudley DA *et al*. Amniotic fluid embolism: analysis of the national registry. *Am J Obstet Gynecol*. 1995; **172**: 1158–67.

9 Fletcher SJ, Parr MJ. Amniotic fluid embolism: a case report and review. *Resuscitation*. 2000; **43**: 141–6.

10 Tuffnell DJ. United Kingdom Amniotic Fluid Embolism Register. *Br J Obstet Gynaecol*. 2005; **112**: 1625–9.

11 Department of Health. *Why Mothers Die, 2000–2002. The Sixth Report on the Confidential Enquiries into Maternal Deaths in the United Kingdom*. London: RCOG Press; 2004. p. 30, p. 228.

12 Atrash HK, Koonin LM, Lawson HW *et al*. Maternal mortality in the United States, 1979–1986. *Obstet Gynecol*. 1990; **76**: 1055–60.

13 Burrows A, Khoo SK. The amniotic fluid embolism syndrome: 10 years' experience at a major teaching hospital. *Aust N Z J Obstet Gynaecol*. 1995; **35**: 245–50.

14 Dib N, Bajwa T. Amniotic fluid embolism causing severe left ventricular dysfunction and death: case report and review of the literature. *Cathet Cardiovasc Diagn*. 1996; **39**: 177–80.

15 Department of Health. *Why Mothers Die. Report on the Confidential Enquiries into Maternal Deaths in the United Kingdom, 1994–96*. London: The Stationery Office; 1998. p. 59.

16 Clark SL, Pavlova Z, Greenspoon J *et al*. Squamous cells in the maternal pulmonary circulation. *Am J Obstet Gynecol*. 1986; **154**: 104–6.

17 Sparr RA, Pritchard JA. Studies to detect the escape of amniotic fluid into the maternal circulation during parturition. *Surg Gynecol Obstet*. 1958; **107**: 560–4.

18 Department of Health. *Why Mothers Die, 1997–1999. The Fifth Report on the Confidential Enquiries into Maternal Deaths in the United Kingdom*. London: RCOG Press; 2001. p. 148.

19 Adamsons K, Mueller-Heubach E, Myers RE. The innocuousness of amniotic fluid infusion in the pregnant rhesus monkey. *Am J Obstet Gynecol*. 1971; **109**: 977–84.

20 Hankins GD, Snyder RR, Clark SL *et al*. Acute hemodynamic and respiratory effects of amniotic fluid embolism in the pregnant goat model. *Am J Obstet Gynecol*. 1993; **168**: 1113–30.

21 Reis RL, Pierce WS, Behrendt DM. Hemodynamic effects of amniotic fluid embolism. *Surg Gynecol Obstet*. 1965; **129**: 45–8.

22 Attwood HD, Downing ES. Experimental amniotic fluid and meconium embolism. *Surg Gynecol Obstet*. 1965; **120**: 255–62.

23 Schechtman M, Ziser A, Markovits R *et al*. Amniotic fluid embolism: early findings of transesophageal echocardiography. *Anesth Analg*. 1999; **89**: 1456–8.

24 Stanten RD, Iverson LI, Daugharty TM *et al.* Amniotic fluid embolism causing catastrophic pulmonary vasoconstriction: diagnosis by transesophageal echocardiogram and treatment by cardiopulmonary bypass. *Obstet Gynecol.* 2003; **102**: 496–8.

25 Richard DS, Carter LS, Corke B *et al.* The effect of human amniotic fluid on the isolated perfused rat heart. *Am J Obstet Gynecol.* 1988; **158**: 210–14.

26 Kitzmiller JL, Lucas WE. Studies on a model of amniotic fluid embolism. *Obstet Gynecol.* 1972; **39**: 626–7.

27 Azegami M, Mori N. Amniotic fluid embolism and leukotrienes. *Am J Obstet Gynecol.* 1986; **155**: 1119–24.

28 Dray F, Frydman R. Primary prostaglandins in amniotic fluid in pregnancy and spontaneous labor. *Am J Obstet Gynecol.* 1976; **126**: 13–19.

29 Khong TY. Expression of endothelin-1 in amniotic fluid embolism and possible pathophysiological mechanism. *Br J Obstet Gynaecol.* 1998; **105**: 802–4.

30 Phillips LL, Davidson EC Jr. Procoagulant properties of amniotic fluid. *Am J Obstet Gynecol.* 1972; **113**: 911–19.

31 Beller FK, Douglas GW, Debrovner CH *et al.* The fibrinolytic system in amniotic fluid embolism. *Am J Obstet Gynecol.* 1963; **87**: 48–55.

32 Uszynski M, Zekanowska E, Uszynski W *et al.* Tissue factor (TF) and tissue factor pathway inhibitor (TFPI) in amniotic fluid and blood plasma: implications for the mechanism of amniotic fluid embolism. *Eur J Obstet Gynecol Reprod Biol.* 2001; **95**: 163–6.

33 Biron-Andreani C, Morau E, Schved JF *et al.* Amniotic fluid embolism with haemostasis complications: primary fibrinogenolysis or disseminated intravascular coagulation? *Pathophysiol Haemost Thromb.* 2003; **33**: 170–1.

34 Levy R, Furman B, Hagay ZJ. Fetal bradycardia and disseminated coagulopathy: atypical presentation of amniotic fluid emboli. *Acta Anaesthesiol Scand.* 2004; **48**: 1214–15.

35 Kobayashi H, Ohi H, Terao TA. A simple, non-invasive, sensitive method for diagnosis of amniotic fluid embolism by monoclonal antibody TKH-2 that recognizes NeuAc alpha 2-6GalNAc. *Am J Obstet Gynecol.* 1993; **168**: 848–53.

36 Kanayma N, Yamazaki T, Naruse H *et al.* Determining zinc coproporphyrin in maternal plasma – a new method for diagnosing amniotic fluid embolism. *Clin Chem.* 1992; **38**: 526–9.

37 Nishio H, Matsui K, Miyazaki T *et al.* A fatal case of amniotic fluid embolism with elevation of serum mast cell tryptase. *Forensic Sci Int.* 2002; **126**: 53–6.

38 Farrar SC, Gherman RB. Serum tryptase analysis in a woman with amniotic fluid embolism. A case report. *J Reprod Med.* 2001; **46**: 926–8.

39 Benson MD, Kobayashi H, Silver RK *et al.* Immunologic studies in presumed amniotic fluid embolism. *Obstet Gynecol.* 2001; **97**: 510–14.

40 Tuffnell D. Amniotic fluid embolism. *Curr Opin Obstet Gynecol.* 2003; **15**: 119–22.

41 Sprung J, Cheng SY, Patel S. When to remove an epidural catheter in a parturient with disseminated intravascular coagulation. *Reg Anesth.* 1992; **17**: 351–4.

42 Clark SL. Successful pregnancy outcomes after amniotic fluid embolism. *Am J Obstet Gynecol.* 1992; **167**: 511–12.

CHAPTER 9 Sepsis

1 Intensive Care National Audit and Research Centre (ICNARC). *Case Mix Programme Database, 2001.* ICNARC data, based on the number of cases identified in the first 24 hours of admission to ICU; www.icnarc.org

2 Department of Health. *Why Mothers Die, 2000–2002. The Sixth Report on the Confidential Enquiries into Maternal Deaths in the United Kingdom.* London: RCOG Press; 2004.

3 Dellinger RP, Carlet JM, Masur H *et al.* Surviving Sepsis Campaign guidelines for management of severe sepsis and septic shock. *Crit Care Med.* 2004; **32**: 858–73.

4 Loudon I. *The Tragedy of Childbed Fever.* Oxford: Oxford University Press; 2000.

5 Department of Health and Social Security. *Report on Confidential Enquiries into Maternal Deaths in England and Wales, 1982–84.* Reports on Health and Social Subjects No. 34. London: HMSO; 1989.

6 Department of Health. *Why Mothers Die, 1997–1999. The Fifth Report on the Confidential Enquiries into Maternal Deaths in the United Kingdom.* London: RCOG Press; 2001.

7 Department of Health. *Why Mothers Die. Report on the Confidential Enquiries into Maternal Deaths in the United Kingdom, 1994–96.* London: The Stationery Office; 1998.

8 Department of Health. *Report on Confidential Enquiries into Maternal Deaths in the United Kingdom, 1991–1993.* London: HMSO; 1996.

9 Department of Health. *Report on Confidential Enquiries into Maternal Deaths in the United Kingdom, 1988–1990.* London: HMSO; 1994.

10 Department of Health. *Report on Confidential Enquiries into Maternal Deaths in the United Kingdom, 1985–1987.* London: HMSO; 1991.

11 Bone RC, Balk RA, Cerra FB *et al.* American College of Chest Physicians/Society of Critical Care Medicine Consensus Conference: definitions for sepsis and organ failure and guidelines for innovative therapy in sepsis. *Crit Care Med.* 1992; **20**: 864–74.

12 Wright SD, Ramos RA, Tobias PS *et al.* CD14, a receptor for complexes of lipopolysaccharide (LPS) and LPS binding protein. *Science.* 1990; **249**: 1431–3.

13 Dziarski R, Ulmer AJ, Gupta D. Interactions of CD14 with components of Gram-positive bacteria. *Chem Immunol.* 2000; **74**: 83–107.

14 Macdonald J, Galley HF, Webster NR. Oxidative stress and gene expression in sepsis. *Br J Anaesth.* 2003; **90**: 221–32.

15 Spellerberg B, Rosenow C, Sha W *et al.* Pneumococcal cell wall activates NF-kappa B in human monocytes: aspects distinct from endotoxin. *Microb Pathog.* 1996; **20**: 309–17.

16 Parillo JE, Parker MM, Natanson C *et al.* Septic shock: advances in the understanding of pathogenesis, cardiovascular dysfunction, and therapy. *Ann Intern Med.* 1990; **113**: 227–42.

17 Taylor BS, Geller DA. Molecular regulation of the human inducible nitric oxide synthase (iNOS) gene. *Shock.* 2000; **13**: 413–24.

18 Natanson C, Fink MP, Ballantyne HK *et al.* Gram-negative bacteremia produces both severe systolic and diastolic dysfunction in a canine model that simulates human septic shock. *J Clin Invest.* 1986; **78**: 259–70.

19 Cunnion RE, Parrillo JE. Myocardial dysfunction in sepsis. *Crit Care Clin.* 1989; **5**: 99–117.

20 Cooper MS, Stewart PM. Corticosteroid insufficiency in acutely ill patients. *NEJM.* 2003; **348**: 727–34.

21 Massignon D, Lepape A, Bienvenu J *et al.* Coagulation/fibrinolysis balance in septic shock related to cytokines and clinical state. *Haemostasis.* 1994; **24**: 36–48.

22 Fourrier F, Chopin C, Goudemand J *et al.* Septic shock, multiple organ failure and disseminated intravascular coagulation: compared patterns of antithrombin III, protein C and protein S deficiencies. *Chest.* 1992; **101**: 816–23.

23 Bungum L, Tollan A, Oian P. Antepartum to postpartum changes in transcapillary fluid balance. *Br J Obstet Gynaecol.* 1990; **97**: 838–42.

24 Peres-Bota D, Lopes-Ferreira F, Melot C *et al.* Body temperature alterations in the critically ill. *Intensive Care Med.* 2004; **30**: 811–16.

25 Smaill F, Hofmeyr GJ. Antibiotic prophylaxis for Caesarean section. *The Cochrane Database of Systematic Reviews. Issue 3.* CD 000933 Oxford: Update Software; 2002.

26 Hopkins L, Smaill F. Antibiotic prophylaxis regimens and drugs for Caesarean section. *The Cochrane Database of Systematic Reviews. Issue 2.* CD 001136 Oxford: Update Software; 2000.

27 Soper DE, Mayhall CG, Dalton HP. Risk factors for intra-amniotic infection: a prospective epidemiological study. *Am J Obstet Gynecol.* 1989; **161**: 562–6.

28 Rouse DJ, Landon M, Spong CY. National Institute of Child Health and Human Development, Maternal–Fetal Medicine Units Network. The Maternal–Fetal Medicine Units Cesarean Registry: chorioamnionitis at term and its duration – relationship to outcomes. *Am J Obstet Gynecol.* 2004; **191**: 211–16.

29 Gallup DG, Freedman MA, Meguiar RV *et al.* Necrotizing fasciitis in gynecologic and obstetric patients: a surgical emergency. *Am J Obstet Gynecol.* 2002; **187**: 305–11.

30 Fernandez-Perez ER, Salman S, Pendem S *et al.* Sepsis during pregnancy. *Crit Care Med.* 2005; **33 (Suppl. 2)**: S286–93.

31 Ogilvie MM. Antiviral prophylaxis and treatment in chicken pox. A review prepared for the UK Advisory Group on Chicken Pox on behalf of the British Society for the Study of Infection. *J Infect.* 1998; **36 (Suppl. 1)**: 31–8.

32 Taha ET, Biggar RJ, Broadhead RL *et al.* Effect of cleansing the birth canal with antiseptic solution on maternal and newborn morbidity and mortality in Malawi: clinical trial. *BMJ.* 1997; **315**: 216–19.

33 Reid VC, Hartmann KE, McMahon M *et al.* Vaginal preparation with povodone iodine and post-cesarean infectious morbidity: a randomized controlled trial. *Obstet Gynecol.* 2001; **97**: 147–52.

34 Subbe CP, Davies RG, Williams E *et al.* Effect of introducing the Modified Early Warning score on clinical outcomes, cardiopulmonary arrests and intensive care utilisation in acute medical admissions. *Anaesthesia.* 2003; **58**: 797–802.

35 Goldhill DR, McNarry AF. Physiological abnormalities in early warning scores are related to mortality in adult inpatients. *Br J Anaesth.* 2004; **92**: 882–4.

36 Lee A, Bishop G, Hillman KM *et al.* The Medical Emergency Team. *Anaesth Intensive Care.* 1995; **23**: 183–6.

37 Department of Health. *Comprehensive Critical Care: a review of adult critical care services.* London: Department of Health; 2000.

38 Rivers E, Nguyen B, Havstad S *et al.* Early goal-directed therapy in the treatment of severe sepsis and septic shock. *NEJM.* 2001; **345**: 1368–77.

CHAPTER 10 Intensive care

1 Department of Health. *Report on Confidential Enquiries into Maternal Deaths in the United Kingdom, 1991–1993.* London: HMSO; 1996.

2 www.ics.ac.uk/downloads/icsstandards-levelsofca.pdf

3 Department of Health. *Comprehensive Critical Care.* London: Department of Health; 2000; www.doh.gov.uk/nhsexec/compcritcare.htm

4 Department of Health. *Quality Critical Care: beyond 'Comprehensive Critical Care'.* London: Department of Health; 2005.

5 www.publications.parliament.uk/pa/cm200506/cmhansrd/cm050526/text/50526w20.htm

6 Hazelgrove JF, Price C, Pappachan VJ *et al.* Multicenter study of obstetric admissions to 14 intensive care units in southern England. *Crit Care Med.* 2001; **29:** 770–75.

7 Harrison DA, Penny JA, Yentis SM *et al.* Case mix, outcome and activity for obstetric admissions to adult, general critical care units: a secondary analysis of the ICNARC Case Mix Programme Database. *Crit Care.* 2005; **9 (Suppl. 3):** S25–37.

8 Bouvier-Colle MH, Salanave B *et al.* Obstetric patients treated in intensive care units and mortality. *Eur J Obstet Gynecol Reprod Biol.* 1996; **65:** 121–5.

9 Baskett TF, Sternadel J. Maternal intensive care and near-miss mortality in obstetrics. *Br J Obstet Gynaecol.* 1998; **105:** 981–4.

10 Wheatley E, Farkas A, Watson D. Obstetric admissions to an intensive therapy unit. *Int J Obstet Anesth.* 1995; **5:** 221–4.

11 Waterstone N, Bewley S, Wolfe C. Incidence and predictors of severe obstetric morbidity: case–control study. *BMJ.* 2001; **322:** 1089–93.

12 Department of Health. Intensive care. In: *Why Mothers Die. Report on Confidential Enquiries into Maternal Deaths in the United Kingdom, 1997–1999.* London: RCOG Press; 2001. pp. 309–16.

13 Smith M, Cooper GM, Clutton-Brock TH *et al.* Five cases of severe cardiac disease in pregnancy: outcomes and costs. *Int J Obstet Anesth.* 2001; **10:** 58–63.

14 Department of Health. Trends in intensive care. In: *Confidential Enquiries into Maternal Deaths, 2000–2002.* London: RCOG Press; 2004. p. 237.

15 Quinn M. Automated blood pressure measurement devices: a potential source of morbidity in preeclampsia? *Am J Obstet Gynecol.* 1994; **170:** 1303–7.

16 www.mhra.gov.uk/home/idcplg?IdcService=GET_FILE&dID=18042&noSaveAs=1&Rendition=WEB

17 National Institute for Clinical Excellence. *Guidance on the Use of Ultrasound Devices for Placing Central Venous Catheters.* London: National Institute for Clinical Excellence; 2002.

18 Department of Health. Deaths associated with anaesthesia. In: *Confidential Enquiries into Maternal Deaths, 1991–1993.* London: HMSO; 1996. pp. 87–102.

19 Young JD. Right heart catheterization in intensive care. *Br J Anaesth.* 2001; **86:** 327–9.

20 Connors AF Jr, Speroff T, Dawson NV *et al.* The effectiveness of right heart catheterization in the initial care of critically ill patients. SUPPORT Investigators. *JAMA.* 1996; **276:** 889–97.

21 Harvey S, Harrison DA, Singer M *et al.* Assessment of the clinical effectiveness of pulmonary artery catheters in management of patients in intensive care (PAC-Man): a randomised controlled trial. *Lancet.* 2005; **366:** 472–7.

22 Van De Water JM, Miller TW, Vogel RL. Impedance cardiography. *Chest.* 2003; **123:** 2028–33.

23 Mabie WC, DiSessa TG, Crocker LG *et al.* A longitudinal study of cardiac output in normal human pregnancy. *Am J Obstet Gynecol.* 1994; **170:** 849–56.

24 Bennet D. Early resuscitation in the emergency room: dramatic effects that we should not ignore. *Crit Care.* 2002; **6:** 7–8.

25 Rivers EP, Ander DS, Powell D. Central venous oxygen saturation monitoring in the critically ill patient. *Curr Opin Crit Care.* 2001; **7:** 204–11; www.ihi.org/ihi/topics/criticalcare/sepsis

26 www.nda.ox.ac.uk/wfsa/html/u17/u1710_01.htm

Index